Making an Effective Bid

a practical guide for research, teaching and consultancy

T0133886

Edited by
Ruth Chambers

Radcliffe Publishing
Oxford • New York

Radcliffe Publishing Ltd
18 Marcham Road
Abingdon
Oxon OX14 1AA
United Kingdom

www.radcliffe-oxford.com
Electronic catalogue and worldwide online ordering facility.

© 2007 Ruth Chambers

Ruth Chambers has asserted her right under the Copyright, Designs and Patents
Act 1998 to be identified as the author of this work.

All rights reserved. No part of this publication may be reproduced, stored in a
retrieval system or transmitted, in any form or by any means, electronic,
mechanical, photocopying, recording or otherwise, without the prior permission of the copyright owner.

The text of this book is for guidance purposes only. The authors cannot be held
responsible for the details or success of any bid made by a reader.

British Library Cataloguing in Publication Data

A catalogue record for this book is available from the British Library.

ISBN-10: 1 84619 030 4
ISBN-13: 978 1 84619 030 8

Typeset by Wordspace, Lewes
Printed and bound by TJI Digital Ltd, Padstow, Cornwall

Contents

Preface

This book is for anyone working in health and social care who is required to, or wants to, make a bid or tender for resources – for money, work, people/staff, equipment, etc., for research, educational activities, or for a new service. This will include academics as well as health and social care personnel. It will help you to develop a greater understanding of how to make a successful bid, and go on to compose a bid or tender with the right ingredients to succeed. So buying the book and spending time reading it should be a great investment.

Many people waste a great deal of time writing bids or tenders that are not successful. Even worse, they may succeed in gaining funding but their plans and budgeting are poorly thought through in relation to the implementation or application of the project or service. That can be a very costly mistake if the funding you gain is insufficient but you are stuck with developing the project or service nevertheless.

So learn from the experiences related in this book. Absorb the tips for writing successful bids, and avoid the pitfalls described here. With practice, you should become more proficient at writing bids and gaining funds that further your work and career.

Ruth Chambers

About the authors

Elizabeth Boath BA (Hons), Cert Teaching and Learning in HE, PhD
Liz is a Reader in Health at Staffordshire University. She has been involved in obtaining research funding for 20 years and has worked as a research facilitator, advising, supporting and teaching health professionals to obtain research funding. Liz's research interests include patient and public involvement and perinatal mental health.

Sara Buckley BSc (Hons), PG Cert Med Ed
Sara has worked in the Faculties of Health and Sciences at Staffordshire University for fourteen years and is currently a project manager for a mix of externally funded bids. Sara has worked with a number of organisations to facilitate and coordinate continuing professional development for their employees. This has ranged from short-course provision to innovative training programmes and formal accreditation of workplace learning. For the last seven years the projects Sara has facilitated, coordinated or project-managed have all been externally funded or have generated external income for the University. Sara has managed project budgets and developed internal and external project costings for much of her University career.

Ruth Chambers PG Cert Med Ed, FRCGP, DM
Ruth has been a GP for more than twenty years and is currently the Director of Postgraduate General Practice Education for the West Midlands Strategic Health Authority. She is also Professor of Primary Care at Staffordshire University. Ruth has written more than 60 books and published a similar number of papers in peer-reviewed journals. She has made many bids over her academic career – many successful, others not – from national and local sources. These total around £2.4 million of funding in the last few years.

Rachel Davey BSc, MMedSci, PhD
Rachel is Professor of Physical Activity for Public Health at Staffordshire University. She has worked for the National Institute of Environmental Health in Japan, the Medical Care Research Unit at

Sheffield University and the Royal Hallamshire Hospital in Sheffield. Immediately prior to joining Staffordshire University, she lectured in the Centre for Sports Medicine at Sheffield University. Her focus has been to promote and develop research in physical activity for public health, primary and secondary disease prevention. This has contributed significantly to the formation of a multidisciplinary research collaboration and she has been successful in obtaining research grants for large, randomised clinical trials and population-based physical activity interventions.

Anne Longbottom MCMI

Anne began her working life in a bank in Birmingham where she quickly progressed to working with managers in assessing individual and corporate lending proposals. Following a career break and other jobs, Anne worked in a local further education college in the Faculty of Caring Services. With her belief that all staff within an organisation should have the opportunity to develop and progress, she moved to work for the NHS to promote learning and development. Anne is now the project manager for the development of the Department of Health's Working in Partnership Programme (WiPP) healthcare assistant toolkit at Staffordshire University.

Chapter 1

Introduction to making a bid

Ruth Chambers

Why bid for that extra work or funding anyway?

You could be seeking funding for a range of reasons:

- to boost your credibility in a defined field
- to enhance the profile of your employing organisation
- out of altruism where you believe passionately in the reasons for undertaking a particular piece of work and are prepared to do it in your own time or in a cost-neutral way
- attracting funding is an expected part of your job – creating esteem factors and enhancing your career through the research assessment exercise applied to Universities
- bringing in business in general
- just because of your interest in a particular field.

If you are successful in gaining funding there will be personal advantages for you, such as:

1 You are an entrepreneur by nature, and bidding for funds for a project or new initiative will be exciting, allowing you to develop the creative side of your nature.
2 The ensuing project or new service will allow you more autonomy over your work if you lead it.
3 Bringing in the funding or establishing the project or service will increase your profile and reputation, and the esteem you are held in by others. This may be a very specific esteem factor to add to your CV to contribute to your career progression.
4 Making the bid or developing the new work will bring career development and extend your experience, adding to your future employability.
5 The new work or service may enable you to build up 'transferable' skills and experience; you may extend your current work to a new setting or sector through the new project or service (e.g. introducing a health service to the community) or gain

new skills that you could transfer to a completely different job – maybe leadership, project-management, fundraising, research and enterprise.

You should be clear about your rationale in applying for the proposal before you prepare the financial budget for a bid. Understanding how much you or your organisation want to succeed in the bid will guide you as to the extent to which you may be able to undertake the proposed work at a loss in order to pump-prime a new field; alternatively it can dictate the size of your profit margin.

So consider whether or why:

- you have a reasonable chance of winning the funding. Rough out the costs of the time and resources likely to be involved in compiling the bid, to get an idea of the magnitude of your initial investment in drawing up the bid compared with the likelihood of its being successful.
- you want to make this bid. As bid-writing is time-consuming and costly, rough out a draft budget as an aid to considering whether it is worth making the bid at all. From a wide perspective, initial losses could lead to future gains by establishing your track record in the field, associated contracts being offered, succeeding in other bids, and knowing more about future funding opportunities.
- your employing organisation requires you to make a surplus to meet its targets, to finance equipment or key staff, to fund research or even to sustain your department/area. Check that your bid will be viable once these requirements are factored in. If making a surplus is a principal driver in making the bid, it is essential to plan your budget rigorously.
- this is the 'right' bid to go for – and what your opportunity costs are. What else will you lose out on whilst you're preparing or completing this bid, or actioning it if you are successful?
- you have the necessary resources to deliver the outcomes of the bid that are required by the funding body. These resources could include equipment, staff, skills, infrastructure, dissemination networks, time and money that you might be expected to have in place already. Without these you may not be able to compete with other agencies that are better endowed, unless your organisation is pump-priming baseline resources with a view to attracting future commissions and establishing a high profile in the particular field.
- your organisation will be seen as 'suitable' to tender or operate

the proposed project by the commissioning body or sponsor. It is usual for funding bodies to request that details of your organisation's trading history and current circumstances are included in the bid to assess the level of risk of your failing to deliver if you were to be awarded the funding.

To help you make the decision of whether to go all out for a particular bid, review your history of success in attracting funds. Set up a spreadsheet or draw up a table with details of the outcomes of your bids for, say, the last three years. Ensure that you have calculated the full costs incurred in writing and preparing them, and add this, along with other relevant details such as the types of funding body, the value of the bid against the actual expenditure in drawing it up and submitting it, and other outputs. Use this exercise to review the various financial costs of bid preparation relative to your success rates, and to analyse other related factors and achievements.

Being clear about your motives and purpose in submitting a bid will inform the extent of the profit margin that you will aim for. If you are ambivalent about getting the proposed work because you're already busy, or you do not need the new work for any of the particular benefits listed above, then you could include a substantial profit in the costing you propose. If, on the other hand, you desperately need the proposed work – to pay for your established team members' salaries, say, or to enhance your weak profile in a particular area – then you may persuade your organisation to let you bid as a loss leader. It might be persuaded that initial pump-priming could lead to more lucrative commissions once the preliminary work has been undertaken successfully and you have become established. Be certain in this case, though, that the opportunity costs are worthwhile.

Undertake a force field analysis

Consider all the positive drivers and negative influences in making the bid while you assess whether it is worth a try. You can then gain an overview of the weighting of these factors.

Draw a horizontal or vertical line in the middle of a sheet of paper. Label one side 'positive' and the other side 'negative'. Then draw arrows to represent individual positive drivers that motivate you to make the bid on one side of the line, and negative factors that demotivate you on the other side of the line. The thickness and length of each arrow should represent the extent of the influence; that is, a short, narrow arrow will indicate that the positive or negative factor has a minor influence, while a long, wide arrow shows that it has a major effect.

Then take an overview of the force field and consider if you can think of ways to boost the positive side and minimise the negative factors. You could do this part of the exercise either on your own or with a colleague or your team. As well as adding more positive and negative factors, the others might notice your blind spots and advise whether you have the positive and negative influences in proportion.

Look at Figure 1.1 for an example of some key driving forces and restraining factors that might apply when you are considering making a particular bid. Some of these will relate to making any bid, others will be more specific to the nature of the proposed bid, the likelihood of being successful, and the extent to which your organisation is supportive of your work; for instance, if the proposal you are making extends a field of work that is central to your organisation, it may agree to accept proportionately more risks and less funding than if the proposed work is peripheral to its core interest. Another example is about the period of time over which the funding spans if you are successful: some commissions might allow you to establish staff on five-year contracts that come to be regarded as permanent, whilst a short-term commission will probably result in similarly short-term contracts for staff employed to deliver the work, creating insecurity for them about their job prospects. Your organisation might fear that it will be obliged to transfer your project staff from fixed-term contracts to permanent contracts under employment law, and withdraw its support for your bid even after you have been successful and the grant has been awarded.

Undertake a Strengths, Weaknesses, Opportunities and Threats (SWOT) analysis

As an alternative (or in addition) you could undertake a SWOT analysis to help you to shape your priorities in relation to making any specific bid, or in looking for whatever funding is available for work in a particular field. You can use this technique to analyse your or your team's capability. Work the SWOT analysis up on your own, or with a group of colleagues. Brainstorm the strengths, weaknesses (or challenges), opportunities and threats inherent in your situation.

Strengths and weaknesses relating to individuals in your team might include: their knowledge, experience, clinical or managerial expertise, decision-making, communication, inter-professional

Positive factors	Negative factors
career enhancement from drawing up the bid, networking with collaborators, promotion in new project team; professional development	long hours of preparatory work

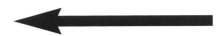

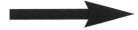

	risks of available funding being too little to meet the funding body's requirements, making the proposed work unaffordable
excitement of having new ideas, stimulating liaison with new contacts	

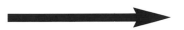

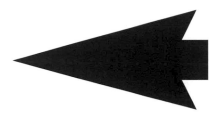

personal and job satisfaction from completing specific task, writing proposal, being shortlisted	own organisation expecting profit; not prepared to 'pump-prime' new commission

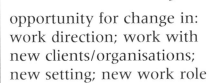

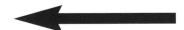

opportunity for change in: work direction; work with new clients/organisations; new setting; new work role	neglect of your everyday work and other priorities

crafting new opportunities for interesting work	short-term-project culture creates insecurity for team members, so high staff turnover

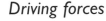

Driving forces	*Restraining forces*

Figure 1.1 Example of the kind of force field analysis you might undertake when considering whether or not to make a particular bid

relationships, political skills, time-keeping, organisation, or their expertise in teaching or research. Strengths and weaknesses for making the bid from your organisation's point of view might link to most of these aspects too, as well as resource requirements for staff, skills or structural items.

Opportunities might relate to unexploited potential strengths, expected changes, options for career development pathways, and extension of your current interests.

Threats will include factors and circumstances that prevent you from achieving your aims for completing the project for which you seek funding, or from utilising the results.

Write your ideas for the SWOT analysis on a single flipchart/sheet of paper so that you and those participating in the exercise can see the items building up on all four quadrants at once. To generate an analysis similar to the example shown in Figure 1.2, ask yourselves questions similar to these:

- Strengths – what are you good at? What factors are in your favour as to being successful in gaining funding?
- Weaknesses – what are you not so good at? What will make success less likely?
- Opportunities – what's likely to be useful in designing the bid that you could harness? What is happening that could help you?
- Threats – what threatens your chances of success? Could gaining the bid generate unacceptable risks?

Prioritise important factors. Draw up goals and a timed action plan. By the end of the SWOT analysis you should be at the stage where you are able to consider:

- how you can optimise and extend the strengths identified
- how you can minimise or overcome the weaknesses
- how you can make most use of the opportunities
- how you can avoid the threats or counter their effects.

What type of funding should you try for?

Where you look for funding will depend on the nature of your proposed work and how ambitious your aims are. Think about why you want to undertake the project, who you will be involving as subjects, what the likely outputs and outcomes will be, and who can support or contribute to the bid. These will influence the likelihood of success in applying for particular sources of funding.

Strengths	Weaknesses
• Will utilise your (you/your team's) knowledge and skills • Have good collaborators in the field of the bid already • Well known in the field/ acknowledged lead in the area • Already have related development work underway • Project staff in place with relevant knowledge, skills and capacity • Good business planning in place with real understanding of what investment is needed • Current resources (e.g. database of contacts, equipment) will give added value to any bid • Sponsors trust your/your team's profile because of your track record of recognised achievements (e.g. your research assessment exercise profile)	• You may need to recruit new project staff with specific skills and experience, or ask your current staff to learn and apply new skills (quickly!) • You and your staff are already committed to ongoing and unfinished commissions • There is poor workforce planning in your organisation, resulting in insufficient staff to undertake a variety of jobs (e.g. statistics, administration) • You and your team have insufficient expert knowledge in the field in which you're bidding • You have limited capacity for the supervision of novice staff, so project staff are not enabled to develop in their roles and take on delegated tasks • There's too little awareness of and familiarity with the commissioner's priorities and issues • A past blemish on the reputation of you or your team (deserved or not) creates mistrust of your bid • You are unfamiliar with the language, jargon or abbreviations used by commissioner
Opportunities	Threats
• The commission matches your aspirations and chimes with your values and beliefs	• Your employing organisation insists on high overheads or profit margins, making proposed *continued*

Figure 1.2 SWOT analysis underpinning the decision about whether it's worth making a bid

Opportunities (cont.)	_Threats (cont.)_
• Gaining this commission will enable you to continue funding the contracts of your current team • Your networking means you know about commissions before they are announced, and have longer to prepare a bid • Knowing the members of the interview panel or commissioners in a personal way means that you already have a relationship, and they know of your strengths and achievements • Your public relations officer capitalises on your being shortlisted (in the event that you're not successful in the end) and any bids awarded • Good links to media help promote your work and your successful bids • Focusing on a niche area that is relatively unexplored means that gaining bids and then publishing the work in peer-reviewed journals should be relatively 'easy'	work untenable within the advertised budget • Your organisation is undergoing substantial change, leading to uncertainty within the staff (who may leave) • Your 'day' job is exhausting, leaving you with too little energy to work up a competitive bid • Your organisation's support services (e.g. finance, HR) are fragmented or barely existent • The bidding document or invitation to tender is ambiguous and difficult to understand, so you cannot be sure you are addressing the funding body's purpose and expectations • You find a sometime 'enemy' or competitor on the interview panel when you present your bid in person • You may have to bid for funding for work that is of little interest to you, just to survive financially

Figure 1.2 SWOT analysis (continued)

Also consider the competition ratio – the likelihood that you will be successful for relatively different types and amounts of funding. On the whole, the more local the funding, the better your chances of being successful. This will be partly because there will be less competition, and partly because you may be familiar with the context in which the funding is being made available and more likely to generate a proposal that matches the sponsor's circumstances and expectations.

Types of awards and sources of funding

Principal sources of funding include:

- Research Councils
- Foundations and Charities
- Government departments
- Commercial sources

Table 1.1 gives examples of award-giving bodies that have funds for health-related research and development.

Table 1.1 Examples of award-giving bodies relevant to health-related research and development

Funding body	Details	Contact details
Association of Medical Research Charities	These UK charities fund medical and health research	www.amrc.org.uk
Big Lottery Fund	Has a range of funding programmes	www.biglotteryfund.org.uk
British Medical Association	Annual research awards from around £200 to £32,000	www.bma.org.uk
Cancer Research UK	A leading charity dedicated to research on the causes, treatment and prevention of cancer	www.cancerresearchuk.org
Claire Wand Fund	Up to several thousand pounds for research or educational study for GPs	www.bma.org.uk
Commercial source, e.g. pharmaceutical company e.g. Roche		www.roche.com

continued

Table 1.1 Examples of award-giving bodies (continued)

Funding body	Details	Contact details
Commission, e.g. from NHS, local government		www.dh.gov.uk www.local.dtlr.gov.uk/ research/what.htm
Economic and Social Research Council	Research awards which offer standard grants £100,000 to £1.5m and small grants £15,000 to £99,999; spent £81m in 2004–5 on new research grants	www.esrc.ac.uk
European funding		See www.rdinfo.org.uk for information about European and other international sources of funding See www.esf.org for information published by the European Science Foundation
Health Foundation	Funds specific healthcare topics. Offers Harkness/Health Foundation Fellowships in healthcare policy – 1 year sabbatical in USA	www.health.org.uk
King's Fund	Supports research in London	www.kingsfund.org.uk
Medical Research Council	Research grants tailored to scientific needs of proposal – budget of £168m in 2004–5 to spend on new research grants	www.mrc.ac.uk

continued

Table 1.1 Examples of award-giving bodies (continued)

Funding body	Details	Contact details
National calls for bids e.g. NHS Service Delivery and Organisation R&D Programme; DH Health Technology Assessment Programme	Fund research on priority issues identified through the Listening Exercise and consultation	www.sdo.lshtm.ac.uk www.ncchta.org/calls/ index.htm
Research Charity e.g. The Wellcome Trust Action Medical Research; offer grants for a wide range of medical research		www.wellcome.ac.uk www.action.org.uk
Royal College of General Practitioners: Scientific Foundation Board	Funds specific clinical topics e.g. cardio-vascular disease, obesity, and any topic relevant to primary care up to £10,000	www.rcgp.org.uk/default. aspx?page=764
The Arthritis Research Campaign (ARC)	Makes annual awards of ~ £20m for relevant research into the cause, cure and treatment of arthritis and related musculoskeletal diseases	www.arc.org.uk
University-funded e.g. via internal development money		
Winston Churchill Memorial Trust	Award can cover travel, living expenses and equipment; aim is to understand the lives and work of people in other countries	www.wcmt.org.uk

Boxes 1.1 and 1.2 contain more contact details for general and specific information about research funding.

Box 1.1 Information sources in relation to potential research funding and the research process

For all calls from national Department of Health and NHS Research & Development programmes for research proposals see
www.dh.gov.uk/ProcurementAndProposals/RDCallsForProposals/fs/en

RDFunding:
www.rdfunding.org.uk/Queries/WhatsNew.asp
or
www.rdinfo.org.uk

For information about training courses, workshops and conferences, visit RDLearning
www.rdlearning.org.uk

For advice, information and support with your research, visit RDDirect
www.rddirect.org.uk

For the research process flowchart, which maps the stages of the research process and provides hints, tips and checklists for researchers at all levels, go to
www.rdfunding.org.uk/flowchart/flowchart.html

Box 1.2 Looking for a grant?

The Times Higher Education Supplement publishes a weekly research newsletter for subscribers online at www.thes.co.uk/newsletters which carries news of the latest funding opportunities, jobs and research.

Academic medical research funding

The budgets of the Medical Research Council (MRC) and National Institute for Health Research (NIHR)[1] (the research division of the Department of Health for England) that fund medical research will be centrally coordinated. The combined funding is expected to be worth at least £1 billion per year.

The research assessment exercise (RAE) that rates through peer review the quality of research in higher education institutions will be revised after the 2008 RAE exercise. The score achieved determines the research institution's ranking and thus the allocation of central research funds. The ranking also confers status, and the top grade of 5-star rated institutions using their prestige to draw in associated funding and support, such as for fellowships or studentships, from other sources. The RAE will emphasise outputs rather than research income, using a 'metrics-based' approach in which effective performance indicators are derived from readily available figures, such as the extent of grants gained competitively from Research Councils, publications, impact, citations, and numbers of research students (see www.ost.gov.uk). The new RAE system will be phased in from 2009–10 in England, and will eventually cover the whole of the UK.

The NIHR was launched in 2006 following the publication of *Best Research for Best Health: a new National Research Strategy*.[2] The strategy describes the direction that NHS research will take in England to build a world-class research environment. One of the NIHR's first programmes concerns research for patient benefit. The programme will allocate up to £25 million each year to fund research that focuses on the way the NHS provides its services and whether those services are effective and provide value for money. The five founding departments of the first research school within the NIHR – the School for Primary Care Research – will be those from the Universities of Birmingham, Bristol, Cambridge, Manchester and Oxford. A primary care research network will be set up in association, to provide support for research.

Research Councils

If you are an established researcher with a regional or national profile working within a prestigious organisation, such as a university department with RAE 5-star status, then you have a good chance of attracting funding from research councils and medical research charities for a substantial research project or linked project within a programme of serious, scientific research which contributes significantly to what is known across the world about your subject, and is conducted in a valid and reliable way with sufficient power to be sure about the findings. You might be the lead, or one of several collaborating organisations, contributing to such a research programme.

Community funds

If you are interested in community development projects with obvious practical outputs that benefit or support particular groups of the population, then you might look at trying to obtain funding from the National Lottery. The Lottery prioritised funding for projects to do with health and wellbeing in 2006, and nutrition, physical activity and mental health were the specified theme areas.

Health service or local government funding

If you work within the health service or local government, or collaborate with individuals in these organisations' workforce, you may hear of local or regional opportunities to bid for commissioned projects. These might include straightforward consultancy, where you would provide a designated service – a review, an evaluation, teaching and training, or development work of some kind. Or you might be one of several individuals or organisations asked to tender for providing a service or project (see page 17). Health and local government bodies are often small organisations without the comprehensive expertise they need to deliver all their functions. They depend on commissioning individuals and organisations to undertake discrete tasks, and by so doing they can limit their core staff numbers but at the same time operate with a wide spread of expertise.

National government funding

National government funding is similar in purpose to local and regional funding, but on a larger scale. This means that the research or development project will be undertaken in such a way that findings are applicable to the nation as a whole, or provide opportunities or benefits to the nation (e.g. learning resources, or a review of national services). Sometimes national funding is made available for addressing important questions, or for conducting research to fill specific gaps.

A recent national initiative has been to develop the UK clinical research collaboration (UKCRC). Those involved have mapped current research across the UK funded by the eleven largest government and charity funders of health-related research. If you look at this analysis of the distribution of funding, you can gain an overview of the types of research fields that attract the most funding, and the geographical distribution of funding. The research analysis[3] indicates that 25 per cent of the total funded research is applicable to all diseases, or to health and wellbeing in general; and 75 per cent relates to specific diseases and areas of health. Cancer, neurological, infection and cardiovascular research made up two-thirds of the funding allocated to specific diseases and areas of health.

Another report *Medical Research: Assessing the Benefits to Society*[4] looked at the returns from government funding of medical and health services research. There are three types of returns – in relation to scientific knowledge, to health gains and to wider economic benefits.

Hearing about funding

Sources of funding are advertised in a variety of ways – in a national newspaper or professional journal, an electronic circulation, a commissioning organisation's communication system, or by the simple method of one of their staff ringing around networks of likely consultants or organisations who might tender or bid. Even when such funding is publicly and widely advertised, funding bodies may have alerted preferred providers so that they can prepare to make a bid. A short closing date for submissions may indicate that others have been warned to expect the forthcoming invitation and have been working on their proposals for some time. They may have collaborated with the sponsors in the field on previous commissions, or even have helped to design the scope and purpose of the current issue of funding and invitation to bid.

Box 1.3 gives a good example of how a well-known research department values its contacts and networks.

Some websites enable you to search on keywords to find a grant. For example, www.grantsonline.org.uk is a lead to funding opportunities in the European Union and from the UK government.

Box 1.3 A good example of a collaborative research department

The Department of Organisational Psychology at Birkbeck College, University of London, 'engages in significant collaborative research and has excellent contacts with many public and private sector organisations, professional bodies, and researchers at other academic institutions. Several full-time research students are funded through collaborative research programmes ... The School of Management and Organisational Psychology is recognised as an outlet for Economic and Social Research Council (ESRC) PhD studentships. Such recognition is only given to those institutions that the ESRC regards as providing adequate levels of research support and training in a research active environment.'[5]

More ways to learn of possible sources of funding

1. Networking, networking, networking with others – to hear of new areas of development, possible niche areas, and to learn of forthcoming developments and priorities which are likely to have new funding and other opportunities. Take advantage of any invitations to social events or conference get-togethers (informal and formal) where you will be able to chat to other experts in your field and get to know potential sponsors or strategists. Read more about this in Chapter 2.

2. Register with agency alert services that will automatically notify you about available and advertised funding in your field(s).

3. Register with agency alert services (e.g. that of your local post-graduate health library) that will notify you of publications centred on your special interest areas – so you keep up to date with the thinking and work done in your own fields in a range of journals that you would not normally read.

4. Become a representative on key steering groups or working parties within your employing organisation, or for a professional or special interest organisation. Once again you will be more familiar with the forward thinking in your particular field, the concerns and the priorities, and be prepared to pitch a future bid to address these.

5. Take all opportunities to get to know other experts in your field – or, more importantly, make sure they get to know you and appreciate your work. Then they may invite you to collaborate and bid with them. This means submitting abstracts to as many relevant conferences as you can afford to attend – in the UK and overseas – and at which you can display posters, run workshops and make plenary presentations.

6. Think laterally about possible sources of funding for your future work. It may be that you can widen your field to be relevant to a different population of users or customers, or develop a new format (e.g. e-learning rather than face-to-face training), extend to include a new geographical area, or submit a previous application that you rework to utilise or developing existing resources in new ways. A level of funding you had previously regarded as being too little to be bothered with might pump-prime, and thus justify, a more substantial project.

7. Develop a group of peers who, like yourself, are interested in making collaborative bids. You might each come from different organisations of the same type (e.g. different universities), or

from different organisations of various types (e.g. universities, healthcare professions, Royal Colleges or independent agency). Then you can alert each other to various funding opportunities that are relevant to an individual or have potential for collaborative activity (see Chapter 2).

Invitation to tender

You might be asked to tender to run a project or service. Then you could expect to be one of less than ten individuals or organisations asked to tender. So this informal shortlisting will increase your chances of success and justify the effort in putting your proposal together – unless of course there is one preferred contender and the rest have been asked to tender only to give the preferred organisation some apparent competition so that their proposal appears to be relatively stronger (and see the following paragraph). The invitation to tender might be run so as to involve you in submitting a simple expression of interest, or an outline proposal with a follow on invitation to make a full bid.

It might be that the whole process of inviting tenders is a bit of a 'sham'. The sponsor might already be commissioning an organisation to provide a service but want to push them to provide better quality, more scope, better value for money. The sponsor may not be sure whether they are getting the best service, and want to benchmark the provider against other possible competitors. But really the whole process is a review of their current provider with little intention of moving the commission, and the real purpose is about increasing value for money and refreshing the service that the current provider operates. This should not happen in a commissioning organisation with good structures and probity – see Chapter 7 for more on this from the commissioner's perspective.

Table 1.2 on page 18 gives an idea of how one commissioning organisation sets out its tendering instructions to specify what procedures should be employed for varying amounts of expenditure.

Sometimes the sponsor will hold a briefing session at which would-be bidders can hear and understand the background to the initiative, learn of any constraints or anticipated problems, and become aware of the sponsor's expectations. It is vital that either you or one of your team attends this briefing session. You can generally ask for more information about the tender if you want clarification or more detail. If you write, email or phone for information and receive an answer, the response to your query should be

Table 1.2 Example of tendering procedures in one NHS organisation[6]

Contract value	Method of tendering	Form of contract	Minimum number invited to tender	Authority to let contract
£2,500 or less	No tendering required	Official order	No minimum	Director of Education Commissioning
£2,501 to £5,000	Quotations to be in writing	Official order	Two	Director of Education Commissioning
£5,000 to £25,000	Quotations to be in writing	Official order	Three	Director of Education Commissioning
£25,001 to £250,000	By sealed tender. Select list compiled for each contract	As specified in tender	All on select list	Chief Executive
£250,001 or more	By sealed tender. Select list compiled for each contract	As specified in tender	All on select list	Board

shared with everyone else who has confirmed their interest in tendering, so that every bidding individual or organisation is in possession of the same information.

Go for a personal award

A different type of funding could be a fellowship or another award. Refer to Table 1.1 if you are interested in obtaining a fellowship that could fund part or all of your working time for a fixed term: for example, you might be working towards a higher degree whilst you complete the programme of work for which you won the fellowship. There are also training opportunities for doctors or dentists who are about to complete their foundation programme training or the equivalent, and are an integral part of their specialty training. They include research or teaching, as academic clinical fellowships or clinical lecturerships.[7,8] The fellowships for doctors and dentists are for a maximum of three years. Clinical lecturer posts are designed for specialist medical and dental trainees with a higher degree, to provide opportunities for further research or specialty training.

The benefit of an award might be the direct funding associated with winning the award, or it might be an indirect gain from your increased profile as a winner or runner-up. Other individuals or organisations might ask you to make a future bid with them, or you might be asked to tender for new money now that the sponsor is aware of you and your prowess. Even going to collect the award can give you new networking opportunities, while you sit with other prizewinners or chat with the eminent personality making the presentation. Box 1.4 illustrates the publicity that two sets of researchers gained when they jointly won the 2005 Royal College of General Practitioners/Boots Research Paper of the Year award.

Even if you are not successful in winning the award, you can still capitalise on the effort you made in your submission. Use the content of your submission to generate a paper in a journal, or devel-

---

Box 1.4 Mental Illness and Conjunctivitis Studies Share RCGP Research Award[9]

Two separate studies, on mental illness and conjunctivitis, were jointly awarded the 2005 RCGP/Boots Research Paper of the Year Award. The papers were chosen for their clarity, rigour and relevance to all practitioners.

The published paper on conjunctivitis found that most children presenting with infective conjunctivitis in primary care will get better by themselves and do not need treatment with an antibiotic. The other winning entry found that, in primary care, patients tended to value continuity of care and willingness to listen and learn, above specific knowledge on mental health.

[The papers were: Lester HE, Tritter JQ, Sorohan H. Patients' and health professionals' views on primary care for people with serious mental illness: focus group study. *BMJ*. 2005; 330: 1122-1128; and Rose PW, Harnden A, Brueggemann AB, Perera RP, Sheikh A, Crook D, Mant D. Chloramphenicol treatment for acute infective conjunctivitis in children in primary care: a randomised double-blind placebo-controlled trial. *Lancet*. 2005; 366: 37-43.]

op it as an article for your local newspaper, your organisation's communication bulletin or a professional newssheet.

Funding from your own organisation

If you work for an organisation like a university or an NHS trust, there may be funding on offer to focus on a new development, such as creating a new technique or equipment, or innovative teaching. Funding may not just be monetary but could be linked to protected time for you to undertake your intended development outside your everyday work. The funding might emanate from a national source and your university or trust is one of several linked bodies making it available; and it might not be just monetary but could be linked to protected time and resources to support you on a high-profile personal or professional development course – e.g. to learn more about leadership – perhaps national or overseas. Again, the benefits will be wider than just the award itself because of all there is to be gained from networking with others, sharing experiences and opportunities, building future alliances and meeting potential collaborators or mentors.

Funding for a dual purpose

Will the funding you attract for undertaking a project (e.g. the evaluation of a new service) allow you to do parallel work? Will it mesh with your fields of interest, so you can publish reports that add to your academic achievements? You must be sure, though, that any additional benefit to you is not at the expense of the work for which the actual commission/funding was meant; and also, that 'piggy-backing' any additional work onto the actual commission does not mean that it is poorly planned or skewed. Work that has not been conceived and planned out from scratch with a blank sheet with resources and capacity to match can be of poor quality.

Is it worth all the effort?

A great deal of effort will be involved in planning and designing your proposal, engaging other people and organisations and clarifying their roles, gathering data to justify the bid, and carrying out a literature or project search to ensure that your submission is relevant and as up-to-date as possible. So you'll need to be very clear about why you want to invest the effort in making your bid. You need also to take into account at this stage the after-effects if your bid is successful – in other words, all the work that you will have to do as a result. Do you have the capacity? Even if you are the leader and will delegate to a team of colleagues or assistants, there will still be a lot of associated work if you are the one who is responsible for the project being carried out according to the agreed protocol, to the deadline and within the budget.

The remainder of this chapter will attempt to clarify these potential after-effects.

Taking the lead

As the leader of your research or project team, you should have a range of generic skills to do with running a successful initiative, rather than just being specific to the nature of the project. Think of the complexity of the project, the uncertainty or risks involved in carrying it through successfully, and the calls on partnership between your organisation and others if the initiative is to be successful. You should develop strategies for each of these areas.

Consider the interconnections between all aspects of your proposed project in relation to its complexity. The more you can integrate the different components of the project, the more cohesive it will be, and the easier to operationalise. You need to take an overview of any assumptions you are making and organise activities to reduce risks through good problem management.

There will always be a degree of uncertainty, and all you can do is try to minimise risks such as escalating costs, unexpected staff turnover, non-predicted research findings or breaches of project protocol by one or more members of your team. This will require you to make balanced judgements, and to think of individual risk strategies. Dealing with uncertainty may require you to think creatively of alternative approaches, or to exercise good employment practices such as team-building and supervision.

You may have to work hard to build up good partnerships – see Chapter 2 on networking. This could include finding ways to overcome different cultures and attitudes towards the sharing of resources or responsibilities, and to accommodate the different priorities between organisations and disciplines. Work to harness the diversity between your partners; that way you enrich the project or initiative rather than create divisions.

Looking after your team

Consider the number of skilled and experienced staff you will need to deliver your vision for the work for which you are bidding. Concentrate on building up a cohesive team that functions effectively under your good leadership in your specialty fields.

Hopefully your human resources department will aid you in appointing staff and maintaining their employment. But if you are the research or project leader you should know about good practice in equality and diversity, providing equal opportunities for your staff, supporting their personal and professional development, undertaking appraisal and personal review, providing fair references, and establishing a work environment that enables them to function effectively.

As the leader you'll want to inspire your team members so that they are committed to achieving your research or organisational goals and maintaining the values for which you strive. A really key research or proposal question with potential to do good will help to inspire those working with you. You may be focused on organisational goals to evolve a high-profile research department which specialises in new research fields or niche areas. Or you may present more focused goals to your team that are relevant to the individual projects upon which they are employed or the services provided by your organisation. Individual team members will have personal goals too – to develop skills in various strands of research methodology, to attend national and international conferences, and to enhance their CVs and networks.

It is unlikely that you are pulling the bid or proposal together out of the blue. Unless you are making the bid solely as an individual, you will be relying on the knowledge and skills of your team, your current resources and your capacity to take on new work. If you want to retain your team and demonstrate how you value them, you need to invest time and effort in supporting and developing your team resources. Bear in mind the ten human resource high-impact approaches (derived from Department of Health Workforce Directorate/NHS Partners/Manchester University[10]):

- Support your team through change – with the funding, new people will be joining the team and/or your current team members will undertake different tasks or focus on new project work. They may feel uncertain about their futures if they have short-term contracts or are threatened by those joining or by the expansion into your new areas. So you should be skilled in change management.
- Develop effective recruitment and selection with good induction, to retain staff who are right for your team.

- Careful planning of your team's make-up and its members' various roles and tasks should make for a happy and effective team. Define lines of accountability so that everyone's responsibilities are clear.
- Train up individuals in your team to be able to take on new tasks and responsibilities.
- Prevent and manage sickness absence as far as you can to avoid having to appoint temporary staff. Encourage your staff to maintain a sensible work--life balance (that means you as well!). Promote family-friendly policies whilst organising their working hours so that they can focus on and enjoy your research or project work.
- Develop and implement appraisal for individuals in your team. They can reflect on your constructive feedback and strive to improve their performance with you and the rest of your organisation.
- Involve staff and work closely with them to develop good relationships. This should enhance your teamworking and their commitment and performance.
- Help to create the environment and processes within your organisation and your own workplace that lead to well motivated staff and boost their job satisfaction. This takes consistent and effective people management – even when you don't feel like it.
- Training and development are key for your team. Your staff are your most valuable asset when you are undertaking a new commission or programme – how could you operate without them? You'd spend a great deal of time and energy recruiting and selecting, then inducting and training new staff, if members of your current team leave. It would be difficult to replace their knowledge and skills, experience and enthusiasm in the short term.
- Adopting all these approaches should ensure that individuals in your team experience real job satisfaction whilst working for you; and that job satisfaction will help them resist the pressures of work and avoid employee burnout, so that they remain enthusiastic team members.

If you are the team leader you have a whole range of roles to play as a good manager (see Box 1.5). You will be the role model for your team, being ultimately responsible for the standard of research practised. If you are an experienced project leader, assistants in your team will be to some extent your apprentices, especially if they are at early stages in their research or project careers.

Box 1.5 Competencies and standards of a good manager (according to the General Medical Council,[11] and generalised for any manager in a health or research and development setting)

- Lead a team effectively
- Identify and set objectives
- Communicate clearly
- Manage resources and plan work to achieve maximum benefits, day to day, and in the longer term
- Make sound decisions in difficult situations
- Know when to seek help; do so when appropriate
- Offer help to those you manage when they need it
- Demonstrate leadership qualities through your own example
- Manage projects
- Manage change
- Delegate appropriately – to empower others, improve services and develop the skills of the people you manage without giving up your responsibilities
- Consider and act upon constructive feedback from colleagues

---

Your team may be dependent for their livelihoods on you and your ability to generate and maintain research or project funding, since this is what underpins their work programmes. You will encourage them, chivvy them on to meet their deadlines, challenge them to achieve their best, and be their critical friend.

As a good manager you will do your best to ensure that:

- Systems are in place to enable high-quality services to be provided by your team/organisation
- Services and care are provided and supervised only by staff with the appropriate skills, experience, training and qualifications
- Significant risks are identified, assessed and addressed to minimise risk in line with local and national procedures
- The people you manage are aware of and follow the guidance issued by relevant professional and regulatory bodies
- All decisions, working practices and the working environment are lawful – in relation to laws on employment, equal opportunities and health and safety.
- Systems are in place to identify the educational and training needs of students and staff so that best use is made of the time and resources available for keeping their knowledge and skills up to date. Training for all staff should be:

 - based on their personal and professional needs
 - available to all in an equitable way depending on professional and service needs
 - based at work if possible and take place in working time
 - reflect multidisciplinary working
 - in an appropriate format for what they need to learn (e.g. e-learning, plenary presentations, small group work, reading and reflecting).

Think of the training and support that individuals in your team will need and factor this into any bid or proposal you are making so that their learning and development needs are identified and met.

References

1 www.nihr.ac.uk

2 Department of Health (England). *Best Research for Best Health: a new National Health Research Strategy*. London: Department of Health; 2006. www.dh.gov.uk/ researchstrategy

3 UK Clinical Research Collaboration (UKCRC). *UK Health Research Analysis*. London: UKCRC; 2006.

4 UK Evaluation Forum. *Medical research: assessing the benefits to society*. London: Academy of Medical Sciences; 2006.

5 Birkbeck College, University of London. *Postgraduate programmes. Organisational Psychology*. London: Birkbeck College; 2006. www.bbk.ac.uk/manop/orgpsychology

6 Hampshire & Isle of Wight Strategic Health Authority. *Corporate Governance Manual*. Hampshire: Hampshire & Isle of Wight SHA; 2003.

7 Academic Careers Sub-committee of Modernising Medical Careers (MMC) and the UK Clinical Research Collaboration (UKCRC). *Medically and dentally qualified academic staff: recommendations for training the researchers and educators of the future*. London: UKCRC; 2005. www.ukcrc.org

8 www.nccrcd.nhs.uk

9 Royal College of General Practitioners. *Mental illness and conjunctivitis studies share RCGP research award*. Seven Days newsletter 2006; June 5–11: 3.

10 Department of Health Workforce Directorate/NHS Partners/Manchester University. *HR High Impact Changes – An evidence based resource*. Leeds: Department of Health; 2006.

11 General Medical Council *Management for doctors*. London: General Medical Council; 2006.

Chapter 2

Building networks

Ruth Chambers

The stronger and wider the networks of people you work alongside and with whom you collaborate, the earlier you should hear of opportunities to bid, and the more likely it is you'll be invited to tender. Being in the thick of things should mean that you are up to date with developments in your field and know of expected changes to national policies related to your area(s) of interest. So you can anticipate the future focus of likely funding – that will be focused on national priorities and problem issues.

Your interactions with others in your networks should be to your mutual gain. It need not just be about collaborating over funding, it could be about sharing resources within your networks to build capital together or to strengthen collaborative proposals.

What kind of networks?

Networks might operate on a local basis, arise from a particular interest area or focus on a specific purpose on a national basis. Some networks are worldwide. The size of the network depends on its purpose and its scope, how it is facilitated and how many members participate in it.

Keep in touch with people who are relevant to your situation throughout your career. Don't just build up a base of contacts who will be useful to you to collaborate with over future projects or when making bids for funding. Think and act more widely – you never know when you and your network of contacts will need each other. If you are just starting out on your academic career, you could join researcher and educator networks in your own organisation, where you will quickly learn how the organisation ticks and get some insider knowledge about how to play the system and make the most of opportunities.

You could become a member of the Society for Academic Primary Care (SAPC) (www.sapc.ac.uk) or another national researcher net-

work. The SAPC's annual scientific meeting provides a forum for networking as well as for individuals presenting their research or dis-
cussing new opportunities. The society provides travel awards and
bursaries to encourage networking at overseas and national conferences. If you are a medic, another organisation you could join is the
World Organisation of Family Doctors (WONCA; www.GlobalFamily
Doctor.com). As well as benefiting from the reduced fee for attending its three-yearly world congress and various regional conferences,
members are also entitled to receive some key academic journals at
reduced rates.

Obtain a list of the names of the participants at a conference
or workshop, and make a note of their contact details as you
meet them. After a conference, there may be enough enthusiastic delegates who share your interest to create a post-conference
network of people working in or developing that specialty area.
You could be the one who starts up such a network – then you'll
be at the centre of developments. You might keep in touch with
one another through an electronic forum with bulletin boards,
video conferencing, by a series of telephone conferences that
are chaired with a semi-structured agenda, or at follow-on
workshops. There might be a practical output from your networking, such as a conference report or book on your field of
shared interest.

The NHS Alliance (www.nhsalliance.org) has many membership networks in fields such as nursing, primary care management, clinical governance, allied health professionals and commissioning. The Alliance encourages members to share good
practice and improve the quality of health services. Their annual conference is attended by around a thousand delegates who
are a mix of health professionals, NHS managers, business consultants, national strategists, academics, patients and their rep-
resentatives. Just belonging to one of these networks will give
you lots of ideas for new services or better ways of working,
meeting like-minded people with whom to work up ideas and
share good practice.

Back home again after the conference you could transfer this networking to your own locality and establish or join a stakeholder
network, consisting of various organisations from the voluntary
sector, and from business and industry, all of whom should be
interested in what you have to offer in the way of joint working or
collaboration from your academic or health base. Box 2.1 shows
some more ideas about networking.

Box 2.1 How can you network with others?

- Join a committee: turn up and contribute to the agenda and discussions
- Stand for election on committees and working groups, representing your discipline
- Make appointment and visit key people for a purpose, either as part of your induction to a new role or simply for networking
- Send reports of your work to others
- Run a learner set for those with whom you want to work; or join a learner set yourself
- Get a part-time secondment to a different setting to meet and work with new colleagues
- Draw up a database of experts for a particular specialty area or purpose and invite them to a preliminary meeting where you get to know each other
- Submit abstracts to conferences and workshops where you'll meet like-minded people, swop business cards and follow up leads
- Gain a key position so that people want to work with you and seek you out
- Find a mentor, or a sponsor in a lead role, to encourage you and make introductions to others

Develop a database of those in each of your networks

Put together a database of potential collaborators and describe their expertise in an itemised way (include esteem factors such as recent publications/income generated/presentations given/national posts held, and their personal details including their discipline or profession, the type of organisation they work within, etc.). Then you can consult your database and consider which contacts to invite to join with you in future to complement the skills and other resources you have available in making a bid. Keep the business cards you collect at conferences; make some notes on the back of the card about why they might be useful to you, date it and store it carefully somewhere you can easily find it. Follow up your preliminary chat with an email exchange after the conference, if that seems to be an appropriate way to maintain contact.

Networking is taxing

Networking takes a great deal of effort and as well as generating lots of benefits and opportunities. If you are unlucky it can be counter-productive. Track the strengths, weaknesses, opportunities and threats of networking in Figure 2.1 and consider to what extent they apply to your situation (see page 4 for guidance on how to undertake a SWOT analysis).

Strengths of networking

- increases opportunities for making links for future jobs, collaborations
- you can build up an intra-organisational database of people's skills etc. for future bidding
- you can tap into others' influence or informal recommendations
- you become excited by like-minded colleagues and more positive about new opportunities
- the network gives you a profile and a badge that declares your interest or confirms your belonging – locally and beyond
- one network can open doors to other networks that would otherwise be inaccessible
- a network is a conduit for you to disseminate ideas and experiences, or appeal for new collaborators
- you can develop real partners for making bids and undertaking joint work who will be true to you throughout your career
- networks may be themed so you can meet specialists in a narrow area, whom you would not otherwise know

Weaknesses of networking

- social interaction and face-to-face meetings can be difficult for some people; they may be at a disadvantage compared to when they're communicating by writing or giving lectures
- lack of time for effective networking; being curt may be counterproductive
- managers may not release you from your everyday work for networking events, considering them a costly waste of time
- networking costs: travel, time (for meetings, email, phone calls), hospitality, smart/suitable clothes
- networking with new or key people may take your energy and interest away from supporting your work-based team and doing your day job

Opportunities from networking

- opportunity to promote yourself in different forums, e.g. may gen-

Threats from networking

- declaring your good ideas and visions potentially exposes them,

continued

Figure 2.1 SWOT analysis to consider the effort involved in networking

Opportunities from networking (cont.)

erate invites to speak at prestigious conferences at home and abroad, or to join boards or high-profile working groups

- may generate additional interest and attention in you
- morale-boosting as you mix with people who are enthusiastic about their roles or special interests
- increased contact with people outside your normal circles, so you build new relationships, hear of new or anticipated funding opportunities, are invited to collaborate or bid/tender; the diversity enriches your thinking and excites you
- challenge to your views, hopes and vision may increase your realism or trigger new determination
- extend your understanding of what is wanted in a bid or proposal; you become more familiar with wider context, underlying influences, etc.
- stimulus to change and develop
- may find role models, a mentor or sponsor who may be a referee for future job or research bid
- may provide time or catalyst for reflection whilst you prepare for networking event, travel to and fro, debrief others afterwards
- could bring benefit from reciprocal agreements with others

Threats from networking (cont.)

to others' criticism, or worse, to plagiarism

- time commitment may be substantial without commensurate payback
- inter-organisational exposure or closer working might reveal your strengths and weaknesses to future competitors
- might reveal your plans or share your intelligence in a way that helps a competitor plot against you or outbid you (e.g. they offer more service for less money)
- good staff may be poached by others they meet, leaving your team bereft
- you may be dominated by more senior people in the network and be forced into a minor role in any collaboration, or in the way that the network runs

Figure 2.1 SWOT analysis (continued)

Box 2.2 Enabling international collaboration: an example from WONCA (World Organisation of Family Doctors)[1,2]

A WONCA report set out recommendations for primary care research practice across the world. The shared approach enables international collaboration across different settings and nations. The WONCA recommendations expect that all member organisations adopt:

- a policy that states that best health and healthcare for all depends on robust research enterprise in family medicine or general practice
- international links for research expertise, training and mentoring
- international ethical standards for international research cooperation, and develop an international ethical review process
- development of practice-based research networks around the world.

Within a network you will need to adopt a 'common language'. WONCA is a good example of network partners from different cultures using a common language in respect of research (see Box 2.2). WONCA's networking and collaboration is built upon international standards for research. A page at their website, www.wma.net/e/policy/bt3.htm, has the most recent update of the Declaration of Helsinki, produced by the World Medical Association in 1964, that provides guidlines on medical research on human subjects. Using these guidelines, it is possible to produce a common research protocol that is applied by research centres in a variety of countries, using the same methodology for undertaking the research.

Being a good networker

If there is someone you want to meet – at an event, say – see if someone who knows you both can introduce you. Or join their group and wait until there is a gap in the conversation before asking them a question. Concentrate on building rapport, being warm and friendly.[3]

Good networkers:

- put themselves out personally in order to build links
- take the initiative
- make the most of opportunities
- present themselves well
- interest other people in their views, their work or their fields of expertise

- are genuinely interested in others and their work
- seem comfortable and at ease in different settings
- appear competent in varied circumstances
- will take risks and tolerate rejection from others
- prioritise networking in their everyday lives
- understand systems and organisations and can generalise from one to another
- keep details of their contacts in an organised way.[4]

Find collaborators you trust and respect through your networking activities. You should be very specific about who will do what in your joint activities, as part of a bid or in the subsequent project. You do not want someone who waltzes off with your data, only to return with the study concluded and written up, leaving little room for your views or other input.[5]

References

1 Howe A. Is primary care research a lost cause? *The Lancet.* 2003; 361: 1473–4. (letter)

2 WONCA. *The European definition of general practice/family medicine.* Barcelona: WONCA; 2002.

3 Stone C. *The ultimate guide to successful networking.* London: Vermillion; 2004.

4 Kenway J, Epstein D, Boden R. *Building networks.* London: SAGE; 2005.

5 Birkhead T. *How to choose a collaborator.* In: *How to get a Research Grant. A Guide for Academics.* London: The Times Higher Educational Supplement; 2005.

Chapter 3

Preparing your bid

Ruth Chambers

Read the scoping document and any associated guidance or information about the bid in minute detail. Consider the criteria for bidding and first check that you qualify to be able to bid. Read it again and again until you are really familiar with all the requirements – even if it seems like a lot of bumph. You need to craft your bid to address the priorities and all the requirements and regulations of the commissioning body (using your sources of intelligence to deduce what these are). This will also ensure that there are no nasty shocks afterwards – when you find that you have to deliver a project or service for which there are difficulties or even impossibilities! Check that there are no prerequisites to being able to make a bid or resources that must be in place to allow the project or service to work that are not covered by your bid and are assumed by your sponsors.

Limit to whom you show your successive draft bids on a 'need to know' basis. Any of your competitors for the same funding will be very interested in what you've put in your bid – both the content and your budget. That would make it easier for them to be 'one up on you'. So don't be naïve, and keep up your guard when collaborating with others, unless you are sure they are not making an independent bid. Use paper copies marked as confidential, and think twice before emailing a draft bid that could be leaked by an untrustworthy colleague. Of course, you could play the system and circulate a dud bid to someone who you think is playing a 'double game', thus sending your potential competitors some false information (and exposing the mole).

Draw in as many collaborators as possible. This will strengthen your bid if your collaborators have strong profiles. But be careful to retain the focus on your intended project if you have to address their special interests or needs as well.

Find out what kinds of bids have been awarded in the recent past by the funding body to which you are applying. Is yours a similar organisation to those that have been successful in the past? If not, why not? It might be that your organisation is outside the usual sector linked to the work of the funding body; that might be an advantage, or maybe a drawback, or even an insurmountable block.

Understand the sponsor's vision – it will be your job to reassure the sponsor or commissioner that they are safe in awarding the funding to you and that you will undertake the ensuing work as proposed. They must appreciate that you have thought of all the eventualities that might crop up to impede your progress, and taken anticipatory action.

Reproduce the wording of the scoping document or guidance about the award and address what you perceive to be the sponsor's desires in your proposal, making it easy for the shortlisting panel to spot their criteria in your bid by using their sub-headings, etc. Think of what is being asked for and assess whether you can meet all their requirements. Consider what's missing from your own resources – and where/how you can fill the gaps. Know what the future holds so that your proposal addresses that future vision, rather than the current situation. Include what's possible in your proposal in terms of technology, your learning format, etc., so that you produce a forward-looking bid.

Consider what resources your organisation can add to the bid as 'free goods'. This might be skills, people, expertise, practical resources like libraries or workplace. Funding bodies might consider such added value as critical to a successful bid.

Is it viable to make this bid? Can you readily meet the deadline, interview date, desired/expected outputs? Have you the necessary capacity, or will you be able to recruit experienced personnel within the timetable of the project?

Your working group for drafting the proposal should be well balanced. It is probably best for one person to lead on all drafting and editing for consistency, with others collecting and feeding in information. Then it needs one or more people to proofread the final draft to spot typos, errors, inconsistencies and gaps.

It takes a good deal of time and effort to draw up a bid, so minimise this as far as possible:

- Build on current work and any previous bids – whether they were successful or not (if they were not successful, you hopefully got feedback about why they 'failed', and know how to remedy it).
- Get lower-paid staff to do the legwork, finding the data you need

to justify the bid, or entering your content on the fiddly application form.

- Invite collaborating partners to contribute their parts of the overall application (you will need to be very explicit about what you need and they must do), after which you edit the overall application.
- Unless there is a good reason to justify moving into a new area, confine any future bids to fields in which you already have an established profile and resources, which might include appropriately trained and skilled staff, relevant databases, prior published work, previous research and development applications (and feedback on these if they were unsuccessful), prior research ethics applications etc., and national intelligence on the future of the field.

Involve users (customers, consumers, clients, patients, students, etc.) in preparing your bid, to try to ensure that the project proposed is relevant to their wants, preferences and priorities, as well as addressing their needs and the sponsor's objectives. The involvement will not only help you to prepare a good bid, but will also demonstrate to the sponsor that you are in touch with the grassroots, so it will be good for you to recruit such users as a norm in your everyday organisational work – they can actively help with any stage in a project: bidding, planning, project management, development, delivery, dissemination of findings, monitoring, quality control, recruitment, etc.

Attend any briefing session about the project or application process – or send a representative who can report back with any formal or informal intelligence or information relevant to the shaping or content of the bid.

Take advantage of opportunities to ask questions of the person running the funding application process to define any areas of ambiguity or gaps in the information pack or the judging criteria that apply to the project. There is usually a contact name given, along with a deadline for questions (so don't leave drawing up the bid to the last minute). There is often a procedure for sharing such questions/answers between known potential applicants or those attending the briefing session(s).

Be exact in the language you use in your bid or proposal. For example, if you use the term 'significant', then it should mean *statistically* significant; that is, it should represent the degree to which the achievement is 'true' rather than having occurred by chance.

Search for what is already known about the subject[1,2]

You will not impress the funding body by submitting a bid to undertake work that has already been researched or developed elsewhere, unless you base your proposal on a critique of what has gone before or been tried and an assessment of their relative strengths and weaknesses. So, for your search of published literature and others' reports of their work:

- Be systematic and rigorous.
- Include all relevant databases – whatever is appropriate to your subject.
- Keep an open mind – to all kinds of initiatives you turn up.
- Brainstorm the different dimensions of your search questions to ensure that you have all aspects covered.
- Jot down your search strategy: search keywords (with alternative spellings), key databases and websites, contacts and informants who might signpost you to work not revealed in a standard literature search or work is currently in progress.
- Organise yourself a tutorial on how to search from the librarian in your local health library or professional association if you are not up to speed.
- Keep good records of your searches so that you can go back and retrieve that paper or report which, later, you wish you had downloaded.

Choose an appropriate method in your proposal

Ideally you would choose the best methodology for addressing the purpose of the bid, that which is sure to be completed to time and will generate the promised high quality service or development, or the most powerful research. But in reality there is often a trade-off between the funding and resources available and your ability to deliver the service or project in as near ideal a state as possible. A methodology with qualitative and quantitative dimensions can be very powerful.[3] Adding a qualitative study to a quantitative one should enable you to gain a better understanding of the meaning and implications of your findings, a dimension which should be useful to the commissioner of the funded project. Triangulation, by gathering data from at least three sources to give a wider perspective on a complex question, can increase the validity of your findings too.

Don't get too bogged down by the detail

Every so often you and others involved will need to take a break from your bid preparation to brainstorm about your progress, and to re-assess the development work or services that you are proposing.

Ethics

Ethical practice should underpin any research. Ethical concepts span:

- protection (of subjects in research study) from harm
- truth and honesty (no deception or coercion)
- anonymity and confidentiality (of patients' details as appropriate)
- autonomy (e.g. of patients)
- human rights (at all times)
- respect, dignity and privacy (for and of participants)
- knowledge and choice (covering compliance by patients; deception and coercion by researchers)
- informed consent.

Ethical practice means that you must seek approval for your research and abide by the protocol, unless for justifiable reasons the research ethics committee agrees otherwise as the project progresses. It means not double funding a research programme without the various sponsors' knowledge and agreement that they are paying for the same work. It means ensuring that any other underpinning research is referenced and that no one else's work is plagiarised. In all of this, as research leader you should be scrupulously honest and transparent, a role model of probity for all team members and alert for any malpractice in others.

The main role of research ethics committees (RECs) is to assess the scientific and ethical aspects of new research protocols submitted to them, and then to approve any amendments and revisions required.[4] RECs should follow up and monitor the research programme undertaken, once the protocols are approved.

Consider if ethics committee approval is needed for your proposed project – refer to COREC (see Box 3.1) if you are unsure. Approval is needed for research where you will involve patients, have access to patients' records and names (past or present), and where NHS premises or facilities will be, or are likely to be, used. If your study is likely to span more than five local research ethics

---

Box 3.1 Sources of further information in relation to UK research governance and research ethics

- Department of Health
  www.dh.gov.uk/PolicyAndGuidance/ResearchAndDevelopment/
  ResearchAndDevelopmentAZ/ResearchGovernance/fs/en
- Medical Research Council
  www.mrc.ac.uk/PolicyGuidance/EthicsAndGovernance/index.htm
- The NHS Research & Development Forum
  www.rdforum.nhs.uk/workgroups/primary/pcinfoguide/
  introduction.htm
- The Central Office for Research Ethics Committees (COREC)
  www.corec.org.uk

---

committee areas, then you should apply for multi-centre research ethics committee (MREC) approval.

Do not disguise a proposed project as a development project when it is essentially research – the sponsors will not be impressed by your deviousness, ignorance, or lack of awareness; and your implementation of the project will be delayed by obtaining research ethics and research governance approvals if you get the funding, threatening your predicted timelines for the rest of the project.

Approval by an REC can be a time-consuming process if amendments are required and you have to wait for successive committee meetings to re-submit your proposals, perhaps attending to explain and discuss your research plans. So it may be a requirement by any sponsor that you have already obtained research ethics committee approval for any bid you are making to them, or have at least allowed sufficient time in your projected timetable for gaining REC approval before you access the funding. The funding body will want to be sure that there are no avoidable delays in actioning the project. Funding bodies will view REC approval, too, as a form of peer review, in that others of standing consider the work you are proposing to do is scientifically and ethically valid.

If you do not have time to apply for and obtain ethics approval before you submit the bid, you should still apply to the REC. Then if you are shortlisted for the award you can demonstrate your commitment and reliability and report on the progress of your ethics application. If your bid is not successful on this occasion you will be

---

Box 3.2 A view of the care that goes into research ethics submissions[5]

'It is a rare pleasure to receive a submission from an investigator who knows his or her subject and how to design a trial, who can convey this with care and consideration, who appreciates the importance of the ethical dimension in the work, and who can engage in constructive dialogue with the committee if a problem emerges. What we encounter far more often are researchers with ropey communication skills whose knowledge of their subject, research design, and ethical principles vary from passable to negligible. Sometimes this problem stems from senior researchers delegating submission to their trainees, research associates, or students or to the sponsoring drug company. But also there exist experienced researchers whose hostility to the process of ethical review is expressed in a slapdash approach to submission, coupled with a confrontational attitude to dialogue.'

---

in a better position when future funding is announced and your research protocol already has approval.

Take your time completing the research ethics documentation, paying good attention to detail so that your application does not have the faults described by an experienced member of a research ethics committee (see Box 3.2).

Research governance – keeping on the right side

Research governance applies across health and social care, bridging the gap between health services and science. It is about enhancing scientific and ethical standards, promoting good practice, safeguarding the public and reducing adverse incidents. If your study should be categorised as *research* and takes place in relation to the NHS in the UK, then you need to gain research governance approval as well as approval by a research ethics committee. Other countries have professional codes and governance arrangements for research; the variation between countries can be difficult to manage if your project spans several countries operating different policies and systems.[6]

So, if your study involves patients, tissue samples or NHS staff, takes place in NHS premises, or might do any of these in the future, you need to gain approval from the research governance committee of the organisation you would consider to be the host organisation for the research.

Find out more by following up the reference sources in Box 3.1.

Managing the time spent on drawing up your bid

You'll need lots of time for successive drafts of your project proto-col, responding to various input and comments from those with whom you are collaborating. Discuss your projected budget with your finance department. Organise an early meeting of the proto-col drafting team once the bid is announced, to give yourselves as long a time for preparation and reflection as you can.

The many ways to manage your time better fall into three main categories, all of which are relevant here:

1 *Reducing the amount of work to be done* by refusing it in the first place, delegating it, or doing less of it.
2 *Doing the work more quickly* by doing it less thoroughly or pro-cessing it more efficiently.
3 *Allowing more time for the particular piece of work* so that there is less time pressure to complete it.

Preparation of the bid will probably be more time consuming than you predict, even if you're an old hand at pulling bids togeth-er. It's common to underestimate the effort. Prioritise your time: be clear about your goals in completing the protocol and the associat-ed work, building up others' support and endorsement. Spend your 'quality' time on the most important or complex jobs to do with preparing the bid. It is too easy to focus on the small, unimportant tasks whilst ignoring the big ones, which just hang over you. If you procrastinate too long the job will be even more difficult, as you will forget your original ideas or what the bidding instructions were. If you train yourself to do the least-wanted tasks first, you can reward yourself with a more pleasing job or give yourself some free time.

You will achieve more in designated sessions of quiet, uninter-rupted periods than in a longer allotment of time broken up by var-ious activities. This is the time for planning, writing reports, or analysing progress with the bid. Interruptions are one of the biggest timewasters, especially if someone else could have handled the problem or taken the message, or no action was required. Even if an interruption is necessary, it may occur at the wrong time, wrecking your concentration or train of thought. Agree rules in your workplace for who may be interrupted, and when. Work out a system (and keep to it!) with your colleagues and others at work for letting others know when you are spending quality time on pri-ority tasks and are not to be disturbed, and when you are available to deal with the queries that have built up whilst you were occupied. Get into the habit of regarding minutes or hours as costed time – think of how much some of the activities on which you spend time designing and completing the protocol are worth, and whether different activities are of equal weight.

Include sufficient time for thinking, doing, meeting, developing and learning. You need to be fresh and creative to produce a dynamic protocol to wow the funding body. You can only manage this in the longer term, with a succession of bids if you factor into your daily schedule the right mix of stimulating work, personal and professional development and networking.

Try to allocate at least 10 per cent of your time for dealing with unexpected tasks. Pulling a substantial bid together with collaborators invariably means that you will have unexpected work to do and pressing issues to resolve.

Wait until you have time to complete a stage of the protocol or the whole of a job. Don't pick up a piece of paper and half-read it, decide it is too difficult to tackle or there isn't enough time, and put it down again. You will have wasted the time you took in deciding to put it off. And if you are in this lazy state of mind you might welcome unnecessary interruptions, and compound the timewasting.

Estimate your project timescale in a realistic way

Using a Gantt chart should help you to make a timetabled plan for pulling together your bid. You'll see that the example of timing for constructing an outline bid is conducted mainly to the times set out. The Gantt chart is a useful planning aid for a project. It can be used to calculate project activities for the total expected duration of the project. In doing this, you and your would-be project team are forced to identify all the activities that will be involved at any particular time, and to ensure that they have sufficient resources.

Work with your team to brainstorm all the aspects you will need to consider in drawing up a particular bid, and, if successful, the new project or service. Then design the pathway in the order in which jobs should be tackled and sustained, so as to achieve a well designed protocol. See the example Gantt chart in Figure 3.1 on page 44. Re-consider any risks or assumptions that you are making, add any new features, and if necessary adjust the timing of any of the stages or activities.

Be realistic when you draw up your timescales. Know how long various regular tasks take you when you are constructing the Gantt

		Week 1	Week 2	Week 3	Week 4	Week 5	Week 6	Week 7
1	Prepare and submit outline research project bid	⊢━━━━━━━━━━━				] ◇ ◆		
2	Consider options and agree project outline plan with collaborators and team		⊢━━━━━┤	◇ ◆				
3	Undertake literature search; find out good practice elsewhere		⊢━━━┤ ◇ ◆					
4	Consult users of proposed service about their prefs and current gaps			⊢━━━━┤] ◇ ◆				
5	Assess resource needs			⊢━━━┼ ◆ ◇				
6	Draw up budget; agree final budget with finance dept.			[━━━━┼━━ ◆ ◇				
7	Prepare research ethics approval, and submit					⊢━━━━━━━┤ ◆		
8	Shortlisted bids announced							◆

Figure 3.1 Example of a Gantt chart: preparing an outline research bid
Key: [ ] Scheduled start/finish;
━━━━━━ Actual progress; ——— Still to complete;
◆ Milestone; ◊ Milestone achieved.

chart for your overall project. For instance, a simple survey of say 250 or so people attending an event might take you and your team 120 hours – including designing and piloting a brief question sheet, processing and interpreting the results, and writing up a short report.[7]

Plan rewards for your initiative

Intellectual property (IP) covers three key property rights: copyright on the use and publication of text, pictures or sound; designs of what something looks like; and patents for inventions. Copyright lasts for the lifetime of an author and for a further 50 to 70 years after they have died – in most countries. Copyright is a complex matter, so consult a text on it if you are including an extract of someone else's work, or want to challenge the use of your own work by others.[8] Most IP rights are protected by statute: e.g. patents are protected under the Patents Act 1977 and copyright (which includes software programs) under the Copyright Designs and Patents Act 1988.

You should agree any IP assignments when you sort out the contract for the new work: who will own the findings of work funded by the commissioning body; who will be cited as an author (and in what order of names) for any work that is published in articles or peer-reviewed journals; who will be recognised as the inventor and organise the patent.

See Box 3.3 on page 46 for an example of one NHS body's approach to intellectual property rights.

Producing a business case or budget

Chapter 5 focuses on the thinking and practical actions you need to work through in preparing your budget for the bid. Drawing up the budget will require you to prepare a business case – the information required is summarised in Box 3.4 on page 47. A business case is 'a structured way that organisations use to systematically analyse projects and to look at how they use their resources efficiently'. You will want to cover the cost of employing project staff and buying out your time to work on the initiative, purchasing equipment, conducting or attending conferences and workshops, travel, office expenses, etc.

Revising and revising your proposal

Try to get someone who has had little or nothing do with drawing up the research project to critique the current version of your proposal. Ask them for honest feedback so that you can correct mis-

---

Box 3.3 Example of the approach to IP rights and other rewards by an NHS body (from Hampshire & Isle of Wight Strategic Health Authority. Corporate Governance Manual.[9])

'NHS employers should ensure that they are in a position to identify potential intellectual property rights (IPR), as and when they arise, so that they can protect and exploit them properly, and thereby ensure that they receive any rewards or benefits (such as royalties) in respect of work commissioned from third parties, or work carried out by their employees in the course of their NHS duties. To achieve this, NHS employers should build appropriate specifications and provisions into the contractual arrangements which they enter into *before* the work is commissioned, or begins. They should always seek legal advice if in any doubt in specific cases.

With regard to patents and inventions, in certain defined circumstances the Patents Act gives *employees a right* to obtain some reward for their efforts, and employers should see that this is effected. Other rewards may be given voluntarily to employees who within the course of their employment have produced innovative work of outstanding benefit to the NHS. Similar rewards should be voluntarily applied to other activities such as giving lectures and publishing books and articles.

In the case of collaborative research and evaluative exercises with manufacturers, NHS employers should see that they obtain a fair reward for the input they provide. If such an exercise involves additional work for an NHS employee outside that paid for by the NHS employer under his or her contract of employment, arrangements should be made for some share of any rewards or benefits to be passed on to the employee(s) concerned from the collaborating parties. Care should however be taken that involvement in this type of arrangement with a manufacturer does not influence the purchase of other supplies from that manufacturer.'

---

takes, clarify any confusing text, firm up uncertainties, fill in the gaps and introduce additional original thinking. But don't revise endlessly; there comes a time when you should stop making minor changes and procrastinating, and finalise the proposal ready to submit it. Or make your last revisions to the protocol ready for action once funding is in place.

Do a pilot study first

Doing a pilot study before making any substantial bid will increase your credibility with funding bodies. You will be demonstrating

---

Box 3.4 Information required for a business case in general[10]

- objectives: what the project will achieve
- options: alternative ways to deliver the objectives
- partners or collaborating organisations
- links to national or organisational priorities
- activity: range of outputs expected
- quality: any changes
- training: what is required
- infrastructure, resources, staffing, etc. needed
- income attracted or generated
- risks associated with proposal: likelihood and potential impact

---

that you know the field well because you've already carried out a recent project in the area. That will have given you insights into what worked well and where the problems lay, insights which you can implement in a new, revised approach, with possibly more resources or collaboration. Major changes in your study protocol might trigger the need for a second pilot to see if your revised approach works any better.

Doing a pilot will show your commitment. It will also help you to be sure that the proposed work is do-able – in the timescale, with the limited resources, and in an ethical way. You might decide not to proceed with making the substantive bid or could try to influence the sponsor to reconsider what they are asking for, using the evidence from your pilot study. If you do undertake a pilot study, ensure that you undertake it outside your intended fieldwork area. Otherwise, the pilot study might contaminate your later major research or development initiative.

Referees

The section asking for the names and contact details of your referees is often at the end of a long application form. So you may have left completing that section until the last, not giving yourself time to reflect on which potential referees would be best matched to the particular bid that you are drawing up.

Think hard about whom you will nominate as referees. The commissioners may depend on the referees' views, especially if they know and respect them. Choose referees who know your track record and will be able to confirm that you are a 'completer-finisher' – which the sponsors will want to hear. Do not risk nominating someone who was involved in any of your previous work that had shortcomings. They may not have forgotten an unfortunate incident in your past, even in the light of more recent improved joint working. Contact the referees you are considering nominating, to check that they are willing to act for you and to update them on your recent achievements. Follow up your contact with a current CV, so that they can keep it by them in case they are contacted by the sponsor – they are more likely to refer to your work in the positive way you have presented it in your CV if they have it to hand. Be sure to include their current details with a choice of contacts via telephone (mobile/landline), email and post in your application form.

Why should the funding body choose you?

It might be worth you considering the game-theory approach. Game theory is the science of strategy, using principles of threat and deception. Before making a 'move', you consider how others might respond and take those anticipated responses into account when deciding your own action. 'To look forward and reason backward you have to put yourself in the shoes, even the heads, of other players...calculating what is going on in other people's minds...while...thinking what they are thinking about what you are thinking.'[11] So if you extrapolate from this approach to submitting a proposal for an award or other funding, you need to anticipate how you, your organisation and your proposal appear to the commissioning body, and what they will be deducing about your motives and reactions in bidding for the funding or work.

If you include activities within your proposal which will mainstream the project once funding has ceased, you should gain an advantage over competitors who do not take such a long-term view.

You could offer the commissioning body a great deal of work for the amount of money cited in your proposal. But take care that you do not promise what cannot be delivered. Do not make guarantees, either, about endpoints that you cannot be 100% per cent sure you will achieve, such as publication in peer-reviewed journals. Suggest a range of outputs that will increase the profile of the topic or area of the project or the sponsors, and that are likely to generate some good publicity for them.

References

1 Dosani S. Tips on literature searches. *BMJCareers.* 2005; 10 December: gp250.

2 Chambers R, Boath E, Rogers D. *Clinical effectiveness and clinical governance made easy.* 4th edn. Oxford: Radcliffe Publishing; 2007.

3 Malterud K. Qualitative research: standards, challenges, and guidelines. *The Lancet.* 2001; 358: 483–8.

4 Pich J, Carnè X, Arnaiz JA, Gómez B, Trilla A, Rod S. Role of a research ethics committee in follow-up and publication of results. *The Lancet.* 2003; 361: 1015–6.

5 Masterton G. Two decades on an ethics committee. *BMJ.* 2006; 332: 615.

6 Shaw S, Boynton PM, Greenhalgh T. Research governance: where did it come from, and what does it mean? *J R Soc Med.* 2005; 98: 496–502.

7 Chambers R. Time taken for a research survey. *Postgrad Ed for Gen Pract.* 1993; 4: 37–40.

8 *Writers' & Artists' Yearbook 2006.* 99th edn. London: A&C Black; 2005.

9 Hampshire & Isle of Wight Strategic Health Authority. *Corporate Governance Manual.* Hampshire: Hampshire & Isle of Wight SHA; 2003.

10 Allen D, Parr R. Producing a business case. *BMJCareers.* 2006; 13 May: gp192–3.

11 Persaud R. Game theory for doctors. *BMJCareers.* 2005; 23 July: gp35–6.

Chapter 4

Developing a successful research proposal: case study example and guidance

Rachel Davey

This chapter describes the process of developing a research proposal that has since been successfully funded by the National Prevention Research Initiative (NPRI).

Background to the proposal

The NPRI is the multidisciplinary UK initiative established in 2005 in recognition of disease prevention as being a major research priority which must be informed by evidence of effective and cost-effective risk reduction and behaviour intervention. It is coordinated by the Medical Research Council (MRC) on behalf of a broad consortium of funding bodies brought together by the National Cancer Research Institute, including:

- British Heart Foundation
- Cancer Research UK
- Department of Health
- Diabetes UK
- Economic and Social Research Council
- Food Standards Agency
- Medical Research Council
- Research and Development Office for the Northern Ireland Health and Social Services
- Chief Scientist Office, Scottish Executive Health Department
- Wales Office of Research and Development
- World Cancer Research Fund

The NPRI has three strategic aims:

1 To provide additional funds and infrastructure support to increase the amount of high-quality research aimed at prevent-

ing the incidence of new cases of major preventable diseases such as certain cancers, coronary heart disease and diabetes.

2 To encourage and facilitate cross-disciplinary collaborations in UK preventative research.

3 To encourage research aimed at risk reduction in communities/social groups with a high incidence of cancer, coronary heart disease and diabetes; explore approaches that will reduce inequalities in incidence from these diseases.

Key research areas

The NPRI was looking for innovative approaches and fresh ideas from interdisciplinary collaboration in 2005 to support high-quality research aimed at identifying effective and cost-effective approaches to reduce risk factors and influence health behaviour, possibly through interventions. These approaches should positively impact upon the incidence of new cases of major preventable diseases or conditions such as certain cancers, coronary heart disease and diabetes.

The NPRI focused on four areas of risk-related health behaviour as single or multiple factors affecting one or more preventable diseases or conditions:

- tobacco use
- physical activity
- diet and nutrition
- alcohol misuse.

Research applications were asked to consider one or more cross-cutting themes:

- Socioeconomic and other forms of inequality in health, especially the 'gap' betwccn/among groups.
- The effectiveness of the intervention, and its cost effectiveness in any eventual implementation.
- The need to identify and address methodologies relating to behavioural change (including: outcome measures; biomarkers; study design, methodological development for naturally occurring experiments) and translation from theory to practice.
- The need to develop better methodologies of assessing and comparing cost-effectiveness of preventive measures.

In addition, it was stated that research applications should have considered one or more of the following overarching issues:

- *Environment*: the wide range of environments within society, e.g. the open/natural, built, work/school, home, transport, cultural, media and political environments.
- *Life course*: both inter- and intra- generational issues and transitions between life stages.
- *Communities and their context*: the differences and inequalities experienced by different social, cultural, socio-economic, ethnic and gender groups, and how this affects behaviour in different ways.

Purpose of the call for research proposals

The purpose of the call was to foster new multidisciplinary projects in disease prevention research, and especially those which would not normally be supported by a single funding organisation.

Notices were posted on various websites and in national newspapers and scientific journals inviting outline applications for research projects that:

- had direct relevance to reducing risk and influencing health behaviours, including the translation of formative research and the development, evaluation and implementation of effective and cost-effective interventions;
- addressed the following key research areas, individually or in combination, within the context of health inequalities: tobacco use; alcohol misuse; physical activity; diet and nutrition, in particular, but not solely, in relation to weight gain and obesity.

There were several stages for applications; the first was to submit an outline proposal (see page 53) in the first instance. Approximately a month was allowed for submission of an outline application to the Medical Research Council. As usual, the tight deadline is one of the most challenging aspects of grant writing, as there is never enough time! The majority of funding bodies will not accept applications that do not meet their deadlines, although some have an open application process which allows applications to be submitted at anytime.

Applications were assessed by a panel of UK and international experts and given a provisional rating (see Table 4.1). Applicants with a score of 8 or above were asked to submit a full proposal, for further review and scoring by the NPRI's Research Board (see Table 4.2).

Table 4.1 Referee scoring system (adapted from Medical Research Council; www.mrc.ac.uk)

	Score

Referees decide whether the application is excellent, good or potentially useful, then use the score descriptions within that band to select a score that reflects their overall summary

Excellent quality research

Exceptional quality	10
Excellent quality – at forefront internationally with potentially high impact; addresses important medical or scientific questions	9
Intermediate – midway between excellent and good quality research	8

Good quality research

Good quality and important research which is internationally competitive, and at the forefront of UK work with potentially significant impact	7
Intermediate – good quality research midway between internationally and nationally competitive status	6
Good quality research which is at least nationally competitive and addresses reasonably important questions. Good potential prospects of making some impact on medical practice or relevant scientific field. Any significant concerns about the research method can be easily addressed	
	5

Potentially useful research study

Intermediate. Between 5 & 3	4
Research plans which contain some good ideas or opportunities, but which are very unlikely to be productive / successful. Major improvements would be needed to make the proposal competitive	3
Intermediate. Between 3 & 1	2

Unacceptable

Serious scientific or ethical concerns. Should not be funded	1

Table 4.2 Board scoring system (adapted from Medical Research Council; www.mrc.ac.uk)

	Score

The Research Board scoring system is based on a score from 1 to 6. The Research Board takes into account referees' initial reports and the applicant's response, and their own judgement. Relative emphasis on quality, importance and productivity/impact will vary according to type of application, and the area of research. The scores are used to help rank applications.

Quality: Exceptional

At the leading edge internationally as regards proposals/   6
track record

Very important (e.g. in relation to disease burden/knowledge of mechanisms)

Likely to be very highly productive and have very high impact on knowledge base/policy/practice

Quality: Excellent

Internationally competitive as regards proposals/track record; at   5
the leading edge nationally

Very important (e.g. in relation to disease burden/knowledge of mechanisms)

Likely to be highly productive and have high impact on knowledge base/policy/practice

Quality: Very good

At the leading edge nationally, often also internationally   4
competitive in part as regards proposals/track record

Important (e.g.in relation to disease burden/knowledge of mechanisms)

Likely to be productive and have a modest impact on knowledge base/policy/practice

Quality: Good

Nationally competitive   3

Reasonably important (e.g. in relation to disease burden/knowledge of mechanisms)

Modest expectation of success and impact on knowledge base/policy/practice

continued

Table 4.2 Board scoring system (continued)

	Score
Quality: Modest	
Reasonably important (e.g. in relation to disease burden/ knowledge of mechanisms)	2
Fairly low expectation of success and impact	
Quality: Poor/flawed/duplicative	
Serious science or ethical concerns	1
Not worthwhile; unlikely to generate new knowledge or have an impact	

General criteria for assessment

The most important aspect of any research proposal is to ensure that you match the funding body's approach to assessment. In this case, this included:

- Fit to the call: the application must address the scientific challenges within the areas defined by the NPRI call for outline applications
- The importance, quality and novelty of the scientific case
- The relevance of the application for multi-agency funding under the NPRI
- The track record of applicant(s) and/or their potential within the field
- Suitability of the research environment
- Value for money
- Ethical considerations
- Cross- and multidisciplinary approaches, including details of partnerships with other research councils, industry and charities
- Follow-on opportunities and predicted long-term outcomes arising from the proposed studies.

All of the above had to be satisfied if applicants were to stand any chance of scoring 8 or more (see Table 4.1) and being shortlisted.

The Research Board then generated scores which ranged from 1.0 where a project is reckoned to be of poor quality and not fundable, to 6.0 where the proposed project is rated as being of exceptional quality and considered to have the potential to make an impact of international importance (see Table 4.2). Read the application and assessment procedure for the particular type of grant you are submitting (see www.mrc.ac.uk) to understand the relevance of each score.

Getting started

Think about the following questions:

Have you (and your collaborators) got the right expertise and track record?

If you do not have expertise and a track record in the identified area of research it would be inadvisable to waste your time in applying, since you would stand little chance of being shortlisted. An alternative might be to join a team of scientists who do have the track record and can lead on the application.

   As one of the criteria stipulated above was that 'applicants should highlight cross- and multidisciplinary approaches', this suggested that a number of researchers from different, but complementary, disciplines were required.

Do you have a potential research idea that will fit into the brief?

In other words, the NPRI wished to commission work with high scientific quality, originality, relevance to all the funding bodies, focused on primary prevention, with the potential for follow-up studies. One good way of collecting your initial ideas together is to write brief notes under each of the criteria. For example, identify main themes and issues in the primary prevention of some of the chronic diseases – in this case, the role of physical activity in the prevention of coronary heart disease, type-2 diabetes, some cancers, and obesity. Ensure that you look into the background and context of the research thoroughly. Link this to government policy; the research funding bodies in this case were strongly linked to government public health policy. The aim here is to proceed more or less deductively from these research themes and to begin to organise your ideas and thoughts in a systematic way. You can then get colleagues involved in a brainstorming session which will help to identify your research questions, clarify issues, think of other perspectives, plan your design, etc.

Writing your proposal

Once you have answered these questions, you need to start writing your proposal. This is an iterative process, and will involve further discussion with any co-applicants. Your overall framework will be determined by the guidelines provided by the funding body.

The MRC provides headings (and sub-headings) to which you must adhere, and also stipulates the length of the document, with guidelines on font, page width, etc. The NPRI's outline pro-forma is the framework for the example of the successful proposal that starts on page 63. Many other funding bodies provide quite rigid guidelines, too, as this makes the job of assessing proposals easier and helps to make the submissions concise.

Section 1: Aims and objectives of your study

Begin your general hypothesis with a brief summary of the problem/issue to be addressed. Make certain you refer to the significance of the proposed research in this paragraph. Then list the *specific* aims: be as concise as possible, use bullet points or numbers if there are several aims. You need to be clear about your aims and that they fit with the given brief as this is the whole basis of your application.

If there are several aims for your proposed study, ensure you can address all of these in the time given and with the resources available. Ensure that all the aims you list in the section on design and methodology are addressed (see below).

Section 2: The need for the study

This is really about the background and significance of your research. It is not a literature review, as is commonly believed. This is where you demonstrate your understanding of your field by critically analysing the pertinent work of other investigators leading up to your proposed work. 'Critical' does not mean negative; it means that you are able to appreciate the salient contributions of other scientists upon whose work your own work builds. You should also outline some of the gaps in the existing evidence-base/understanding. Ensure that you state clearly the originality and significance of your proposed work. The reviewers will be looking for what the potential impact of your research will be on the disease or health issue in question.

Section 3: The proposed research

The research design and methodology section is a vital part of your application. A clear statement of the overall approach helps to orient the reader, and will lead naturally into the description of the study design. The purpose of this section is to explain how you will achieve your specific aims.

Novice scientists are often confused about the distinction between design and methods, leading them to lump the two together. Discuss them separately. The design is the way in which you conceptualise your study or experiments, whereas the methodology is a detailed description of exactly what you will do and how you will do it. You may need to justify why you have chosen a particular study design.

The design connects the research questions to the data. Therefore, an effective way of organising this section is under the specific means by which each aim will be met. Begin the section with a brief description of your overall approach, and then describe the experiments to be conducted to achieve each of the objectives in a logical fashion.

The methodology is relatively straightforward, but needs to be written with a critical approach. Make sure you provide your reviewers with sufficient detail to evaluate your proposed work. You may need to refer to methods used by other researchers in the field, or you may be proposing to develop a new method or a new technique. You might highlight previous pilot work you have done (it helps your case if this is already published).

The research design and methods section should include a section on data analysis. This should not simply consist of the names of the statistical tests to be performed, but should convey what types of data will be recorded, how they will be analysed, and what they will mean in terms of your hypotheses. The absence of a detailed data analysis section in a project proposal is one of the most frequent criticisms made by reviewers. If your analysis is complex, you may wish to include a statistician among your investigators.

Another important part of this section is a discussion of the potential limitations of your proposed work, as well as your plans for dealing with them (contingency plans). This discussion often focuses on problems of interpretation. You will not wish to discuss problems for which you have no potential solutions. Rather, you should discuss any technical problems that may arise and what alternate plans you could implement. This is a sophisticated part of the proposal, which should be reviewed carefully with an experienced mentor. Be careful not to be too negative here, and, where there are limitations in your research, try to provide ways in which you will to try to minimise these.

This section should include:

- the sampling/recruitment strategy (and timescale)
- how big the sample needs to be, and why

- inclusion/exclusion criteria
- what outcome measures/instruments you will use (enhancing reliability/validity)
- data collection and management.

You may indicate in the section any ethical issues to consider, depending on the structure of the pro-forma.

End the research design and methodology section with a time-table containing information about how long you expect each part of the study will take. Convey that your proposed work is do-able in the predicted timescale, and that you have developed a logical plan and a competent research team for carrying the work out.

The abstract

The abstract appears at the beginning of the research, but it is presented last here because it really should be written after you have finished drafting the rest of the research plan. This is because an abstract should reflect the contents of the entire application presented in the order in which they appear within the application.

The abstract should be capable of acting as a 'standalone' piece, because it may be the only part of the application that some reviewers read. Consequently, it should be revised until it is a well-written, accurate summary of the entire proposal. Novice investigators are sometimes reluctant to include the aims of the research study in their abstract, since they also appear early in the proposal. But do include them in both the abstract and main body of the research plan. The abstract should also include an overview of the methodology.

Review the application

Review your first draft and go through the funding body's checklist to see if all their criteria have been addressed sufficiently. Try to get some of your colleagues to do this independently.

One of the most challenging aspects of submitting a proposal is meeting the deadlines. If you miss the deadline, all that hard work and effort is wasted as your proposal will probably not even be considered. Meeting deadlines causes much stress, especially if you are relying on a number of colleagues to contribute, who may well be very busy with other things. You don't want to be up all the night before the deadline, because tiredness leads to mistakes. Try to allow sufficient time for last-minute changes or amendments, and to ensure that you fulfil the procedures for submission. Some funding bodies require online submissions, others postal delivery (or sometimes both of these).

The submission checklist

Use the checklist (see Box 4.1) to be sure that you have included all necessary details in your research proposal.

Conclusion

Obtaining funding is an extremely competitive process. Even if you are able to address all that is required, the reality is that there are no guarantees of securing funding. If your application does not receive a fundable priority score (see Tables 4.1 and 4.2) it is disappointing, but do not be unduly discouraged.

Many investigators need to revise their applications prior to receiving funding. This is as true of established professors as it is of those just starting out. The 'trick' to getting funding for a revised application is to be responsive to the criticisms made by the reviewers. This is not to say that you must necessarily incorporate every one of their suggestions into your revised proposal, but you will probably need to incorporate the majority in order to receive funding. It is essential to address every criticism, no matter how small it seems.

Demonstrate that you have considered the criticisms made, and if you cannot incorporate the suggestions, explain your reasons for not doing so. But do not ignore what you consider to be a trivial criticism, as your reviewer obviously thought it important enough to make it.

The tone of your response should be objective, and neither angry nor obsequious. Demonstrate your continued progress in a revised application. In other words, show your reviewers that you are sufficiently committed to the project that you continued to work on it, even without outside funding.

While it is frustrating to have to redraft an application, many revised applications are successful. Keep at it, and the odds are that you will succeed.

Further details of the NPRI and the grants that were awarded in the call for research associated with this case study can be found at: www.mrc.ac.uk/OurResearch/NationalPreventionResearch Initiative/index.htm

---

Box 4.1 Proposal checklist

1 Importance

- Is research in this area needed?
- How important are the questions or gaps in knowledge that are being addressed? Is there a good rationale for pursuing these? Is success likely to lead to significant new understanding?
- Does the proposal realistically set out the ultimate potential benefits with respect to improving human health?
- How important is it to do the work now?
- Is there similar or complementary research underway elsewhere? Is the proposal competitive?

2 Scientific potential

2.1 Environment and people

- Are the applicants able to deliver the work, and keep to time?
- If the proposal embarks on work in a field new to the applicants, or is a first funding application, is there a firm foundation to take the work forward?
- How well does the work fit with other relevant research pursued by the applicants?
- Has the host institution demonstrated a commitment to supporting the work?

2.2 Research plans

- How innovative are the proposals?
- Are the experimental plans realistic given the aims of the research and the resources?
- Are the methods and study designs competitive with the best in the field?
- Have major scientific, technical or organisational challenges been identified, and will they be tackled well?

3 Justification of resources requested

- Are the requested resources clearly justified?

4 Ethical and other implications

- Is the work ethically acceptable?
- Are there any ethical issues that need separate consideration?
- Are the ethical review and research governance arrangements clear and acceptable?

Appendix to Chapter 4:
Outline proposal for the case study submitted to the National Prevention Research Initiative (NPRI)

1 Identifiers and Abstract

1.1 Full title of research proposal

An ecological approach to promoting health-enhancing physical activity in a deprived inner-city population.

1.2 Principal applicant

Dr Rachel Davey, Reader in Physical Activity and Public Health, Faculty of Health, Staffordshire University
Phone: FAX: E-mail:

1.3 Type of funding and period of funding requested

Pilot studies, environmental mapping and targeted intervention: 5 years

1.4 Abstract of research proposal (100 words maximum)

A multi-factorial, multi-agency approach to increasing physical activity (PA) in a deprived inner-city community is proposed. Multiple PA interventions, each based on best available evidence and making use of information derived from environment and health mapping, will be carried out in targeted intervention neighbourhoods over two years. Matched local neighbourhood areas will act as controls. The study will use a cluster RCT approach and is designed to detect a 10% increase in the proportion of the population physically active at the end of the intervention. Participants will be flagged for longer-term follow-up of incidence of major diseases.

1.5 Lay abstract of research proposal (100 words maximum)

Increasing population PA is a high priority for improved public health. There is convincing research evidence of ways to increase PA, yet population PA levels continue to decline and overweight and obesity continue to rise. In this research, we propose to integrate best practice from research evidence across public, voluntary and private service providers to increase PA in deprived inner-city parts of Stoke-on-Trent. Changes in the intervention areas will be compared with matched non-intervention areas at the end of the two year intervention, with an expected 10% increase in the proportion of the population that is physically active.

2 Need for the study

2.1 What is/are the key research area/s to be addressed?

Physical inactivity in a deprived inner-city community.

2.2 What are the aims and objectives of the study?

The study has three aims:

1 **Pilot studies** To develop tools and procedures to reduce levels of inactivity within a deprived inner-city community.
2 **Geo-code mapping (Geographical Information System, GIS)** To conduct a city-wide (for Stoke-on-Trent (SoT)) mapping of the environment in relation to: (i) resources to support PA (leisure centres; sport and recreation facilities and clubs; parks and green spaces; community centres and neighbourhoods); (ii) health indicators (major diseases where physical inactivity is an established risk factor: coronary heart disease, diabetes, obesity, some cancers); and (iii) levels of PA.
3 **Targeted intervention** To evaluate the effectiveness and cost-effectiveness of an ecologically-based intervention to promote uptake and maintenance of PA in a targeted inner-city population.[1]

Within these aims the study will have the following specific objectives:

1 To obtain estimates of the proportions of the target population in the following categories of PA: (i) meeting national targets or at a level of fitness implying adequate level of PA to promote better health; (ii) some regular activity but not enough to maintain health; and (iii) little or no regular PA.
2 To provide an 'environment and health' map for Stoke-on-Trent.
3 To test the relationship between health, PA and higher-level environmental determinants such as neighbourhood socio-economic circumstances, convenience of facilities or spaces suitable for PA, neighbourhood connectivity, population density, land-use mix, mass transport, area social capital, perceptions of traffic and safety (and crime) and perceptions of the local weather.

4 To develop resources, protocols and activities for an ecological intervention to increase levels of PA across an inner-city community.
5 To evaluate the effectiveness and cost-effectiveness of such an approach to increase 'population' PA.

2.3 What are the detailed research questions to be addressed or the hypotheses to be tested?

1 To estimate proportion of the target population achieving recommended levels of PA to within ±5% with 95% confidence.
2 To test the hypothesis that levels of PA and the prevalence of major health risks and diseases are associated with higher-level environmental factors. Specific hypotheses to be tested will be of the form Factor x will be positively associated with level of PA or Factor x will be negatively associated with health risk y. Factors (x) to be considered are those outlined in section 2.2, under objective 3. Health risks (y) are overweight/obesity and the prevalence of major diseases: coronary heart disease, diabetes, osteoarthritis, cancer.
3 To test the hypothesis that an eco-environmental approach to community behaviour change (whereby multiple agencies (public, voluntary and private) and key people within the target community work collectively to achieve beneficial change in a given factor) can increase the proportion of the target population who are physically active by 10% over current levels. It is anticipated that the eco-environmental approach would be iterative and that further beneficial changes would occur across time but that, in the proposed project, the 10% gain in PA would be made up of those who are modestly active who change to meet recommended levels and those who are currently inactive who take up some regular activity.

2.4 Why is the study needed now?

The need to improve population levels of PA has been well documented in a number of major studies[2-4] and in the public health White Paper.[5]

2.5 Has a systematic review been carried out and what were the findings?

A recent systematic review of the effectiveness of public health

interventions for increasing PA[6] identified common attributes of successful interventions but concluded that the evidence base for policy recommendations in the UK remains sparse. Virtually all of the
interventions considered in this review targeted the individual and
were limited to a specific setting. It was conceded by the report's
authors that such intervention, at its very best, will have a limited
impact on population PA and that research and evaluation of population-based approaches, such as that proposed here, is needed.

We have been unable to find any systematic reviews on the cost-
effectiveness of PA-based public health interventions, probably
because of the poor evidence base on cost-effectiveness evaluations
for this type of intervention.

2.6 How will the results of this study be used?

Depending on the outcomes of the project, there is considerable
potential for impact on urban design and neighbourhood renewal,
the development of public health partnership, particularly between
leisure and recreation services, social services and primary care
trusts (PCTs), and on the cost-effective delivery of healthcare services i.e. towards the more 'fully-engaged' public health scenario as
envisaged by the Wanless report.[7]

2.7 What is the public health policy relevance of the study?

The study would make a direct contribution to achieving targets
under a number of National Service Frameworks (coronary heart
disease, older people, diabetes, mental health, cancer, children).
Promoting PA is an important cross-cutting theme under a number
of government policies (Departments of Health; Culture, Media &
Sport; Education & Skills; Transport). By involving the community
more directly in the evolution of its own health, the project should
make a contribution towards a more equitable distribution of
resources (and, thereby, a population more fully engaged in pre-
serving its own health).

3 The proposed research and relevance to NPRI

3.1 Why is the proposed study especially relevant to multi-agency funding?

Multi-agency collaboration is fundamental to the approach proposed. Collaboration between public service bodies (e.g. leisure and

recreation services, social services and healthcare providers) and the target community is built into the design and delivery of the intervention. In effect, these resources are re-directed within the community so as to reset the balance between the factors predisposing an individual to adopt a negative health behaviour (e.g. being physically inactive) to those that predispose an individual to adopt healthier behaviour (e.g. being physically active).

3.2 In what sense(s) is the study multidisciplinary?

A multidisciplinary team of investigators has been assembled to develop the project design, including those with previous experience of large-scale population approaches to PA promotion, GIS mapping and analysis, public health, health technology assessment, health economics, statistics and health psychology. In addition, a multidisciplinary, multi-sectoral approach will be taken to deliver the targeted intervention.

3.3 What is the proposed study design?

The proposed study is designed around three phases: (i) pilot studies; (ii) GIS mapping; and (iii) targeted intervention. The preparatory phases (i) and (ii) will proceed in parallel over 18 months, the intervention will run over a further 2½ years and evaluation of effectiveness and cost-effectiveness will require a further year of analysis and follow-up. The proposed approaches to deliver the five specific objectives outlined in section 2.2 are summarised in Table 4.3.

Table 4.3 Summary of study design

Descriptor	Design
1 Estimate population proportions in PA categories baseline and follow-up	Independent survey
2 Health and lifestyle mapping	GIS
3 Test higher level determinants	Hierarchical Linear Modelling
4 Develop resources, protocols & activities	Individual and environmental
5 a) Effectiveness and b) cost-effectiveness of PA intervention	a) Cluster randomised controlled trials (RCTs) b) NICE

3.4 Are you developing new research methods, and if so, what are they?

No new research methods are proposed in this study. However, the proposed hierarchical linear modelling[8] and social ecology approaches to public health intervention have not yet been rigorously tested in the UK.

3.5 Are consumer or patient groups, other beneficiaries of the research or the public in general, involved in a consultative manner in the development and/or operation of the study?

Local community groups have been involved in the study design. Members of consumer groups, patient groups and the general public will be integrally involved in the development and operation of the study.

3.6 Are there planned interventions, and if so, what are they?

The essence of the ecological approach that sets it apart from other approaches is that what is actually being 'treated' is the area and not the individual *per se*. More precisely, the balance of factors within the community that predispose adoption of unhealthy behaviours and those that predispose adoption of more healthy behaviours is manipulated in favour of the latter. It will not be feasible to evaluate, with full rigour, all of the individual elements that make up this multi-factorial, multi-agency approach, in which several smaller components are combined to yield an overall effect. Where we are able to do so, we have designed the programme element with sufficient power to detect expected differences in the study populations, in the main using cluster RCT methodology. Where this has not been possible, we believe that direct measurement of usage provides a useful proxy measure of impact. See Table 4.4.

3.7   What are the proposed methods for addressing any potential confounding factors, if relevant?

There are numerous potential confounders with respect to population PA, e.g. other PA initiatives, major re-development, re-employment or job loss. The proposed interventions will be taking place within an environment that is constantly in flux. In order to be able to attribute change to the intervention programme, we propose to

Table 4.4 Planned interventions

Programme element and implementation	Evaluation
Walking/cycling: Marked and themed trails; led by activity groups or volunteers supported by maps, 'how to' leaflets, etc.	Attendance (organised events); trail usage; item in follow-up survey
Exercise referral: GP referral supported by leisure services and local neighbourhood redesign	Uptake and adherence; health-related quality of life (QoL) section in follow-up survey
Sports, inc. street sport: Indoor and outdoor activities supported by local clubs, neighbourhood competitions/leagues	Attendance at sessions; item in follow-up survey
Pastimes, active leisure: Link to and promote existing activities; sessional activities (e.g. exercise to music, bowls, dance, yoga, martial arts, Tai Chi)	Item on leisure activities and change in leisure activities in follow-up survey
Water activities: Swimming, aquarobics and 'water therapy' sessions offered at local pools	Session attendance; cluster RCT; follow-up survey
School-based activities: After-school activity clubs: i.e. dance, sports, fitness and health	Cluster RCT

use a cluster RCT design, wherein local areas (natural neighbour-hoods) receiving the intervention will be matched by similar local areas not receiving the intervention.[9]

3.8 What are the proposed criteria for including/excluding study participants, if relevant?

Given the population-based nature of the project, inclusion will be maximised and exclusion criteria will be kept to a minimum. The latter will include those who may be at increased risk from the intervention or whose condition or behaviour may affect the conduct of the project. Minimum age for inclusion will be seven years of age. There will be no upper limit.

3.9 What is the planned recruitment rate, if relevant?

The size of the population included in the intervention and control areas will be ~10,000 individuals (each area). In order to achieve programme objectives we estimate that we will need to recruit approximately 600 participants in each arm (the study panel). Based on our previous study involving PA,[10] we have planned for a staggered recruitment rate of 300 participants per quarter.

3.10 What is the proposed sample size, if relevant?

See Tables 4.5 and 4.6 for sample size.

Table 4.5 Sample required to test main outcome – difference of 10% in population proportions physically active ($p < 0.05$, 2-sided, power = 0.8)

Starting sample proportion	0.2	0.3	0.5
Addresses selected for interview	593	712	771
Minus ineligible addresses (12%)	522	627	678
Completed interviews at both survey waves (60%)	313	376	407

Table 4.6 Sample sizes for embedded cluster RCTs for ($p < 0.05$, 2-sided, power = 0.8)

Study	Cluster size	Number of clusters	Intraclass correlat-ion	Effect size
Neighbourhood (main analysis)	120	10	0.01	0.25
Water exercise	25	17	0.01	0.33
Schools-based PA	15	42	0.01	0.3

3.11 What types of analysis, including any subgroup analysis, are proposed?

Chi-squared analysis will be used to test for differences in the distributions of PA categories in the intervention and control areas. Hierarchical linear modelling (HLM) will be used to examine associations between community characteristics, PA behaviour and health indices. Multi-layer (GIS) mapping and analysis will be used to explore spatial relationships between the environment, health and health behaviours and to prioritise and plan the interventions. Major health events (cardiovascular disease, obesity, type 2 diabetes, cancer, mortality) will be recorded to enable comparison of risk in the study populations over time using life-table and proportional hazards analysis. [NB requires follow-up beyond proposed study period and not costed in proposal.]

3.12 What are the proposed outcome measures (primary and secondary)?

The primary outcome measure is the proportion of those in the target population who are physically active post-intervention. Incremental cost-effectiveness ratio and its 95% confidence interval (from non-parametric bootstrap sampling) and cost-effectiveness acceptability curves are the primary measures for the cost-effectiveness analysis.

3.13 Will the study include any economic evaluation? How will cost-effectiveness of any proposed intervention be evaluated?

Cost-effectiveness analysis will be included under the National Institute of Health and Clinical Excellence (NICE) framework. The EuroQol and the SF-12 will be used to derive utility estimates of effect. Marginal costs for the delivery of the intervention and associated healthcare costs for both intervention and control groups will be obtained from individual diaries and healthcare records. Extrapolation beyond the study period will be undertaken using different cost–benefit scenarios (appropriately discounted) and assumptions on adherence.

3.14 Will the study include any quality-of-life evaluation?

Quality-of-life measures EuroQol-5D and the SF12 and associated utility derivatives (using time trade-off) will be used within the cost-effectiveness analysis. Social capital items (a proxy for quality of the living environment) will be included in the follow-up survey analysis. Lifestyle behaviours and attitudes to healthy lifestyle choices will be included in survey questions.

3.15 What are your plans, if relevant, for obtaining ethical approval and addressing issues of research governance? Are any particular problems anticipated?

We will seek full local research ethics committee approval for the study. At least one research governance lead of a local primary care trust will be a member of the project steering committee. No particular problems are anticipated.

4 Details of study group

4.1 PIs and collaborators

4.2 Other partners and contributors to the project

Should we be invited to submit a full application, a wide range of key partners in Stoke-on-Trent will be involved and consulted in shaping the final bid.

References

1 Stokols D. Social ecology and behavioural medicine: implications for training, practice and policy. *Behavioral Medicine.* 2000; 26(3): 129–38.

2 United States Department of Health and Human Services. *Physical activity and health: a report of the surgeon general.* Atlanta: USDHSS; 1996.

3 World Health Organisation. *Global Strategy on Diet, Physical Activity and Health* 2004 www.who.int/dietphysicalactivity/publications

4 Chief Medical Officer. *At least five a week: evidence on the impact of physical activity and its relationship to health.* London: DH; 2004.

5 Department of Health. *Choosing health: making health choices easier.* London: DH; 2004.

6 Hillsdon M, Foster C, Naidoo B, Crombie H. *Effectiveness of public health interventions for increasing physical activity among adults.* Evidence briefing. London: Health Development Agency; 2004.

7 Wanless D. *Securing good health for the whole population.* Final report to HM Treasury. London: HMSO; 2004.

8 Raudenbush SW. *Hierarchical Linear Models: Applications and data analysis methods.* London: SAGE; 2002.

9 Raudenbush SW. Statistical analysis and optimal design for cluster randomised trials. *Psychological Methods.* 1997; 2: 173–85.

10 Heffron M, Cochrane T, Davey R. *Burngreave in Action: a community approach to promoting physical activity.* London: Health Education Authority; 1998.

Chapter 5

Preparing the budget

Sara Buckley

Work with your finance department or manager to agree the percentage that the organisation will charge for overheads (maybe less if you are pump-priming or working off-site), the desired percentage profit, office expenses and necessary expenses such as for travel, library costs, printing and postage. Include funding for staff development. Allow for additional activities if things go wrong, e.g. staff sickness absence, or if any project activity is postponed or fails. Treat each individual bid separately when calculating or agreeing the budgets.

Why do you want to bid for that funding?

The various reasons as to why you are keen to obtain funding will include:

- You are an entrepreneur by nature and bidding for funds for a project or new initiative will be exciting, allowing you to develop the creative side of your nature with a newly funded programme.
- The ensuing project or new service will allow you more autonomy over your work if you lead or establish it.
- Bringing in the funding or establishing the project or service will increase your profile and build up esteem from others. This may be a very specific esteem factor to add to your CV to contribute to your career development, aiding your promotion to a more senior post or adding to your transferable skills for a new type of post.
- Making the bid or developing the new work will extend your experience and future employability.
- The new work or service may enable you to build up transferable skills and experience; you may extend your current work to a new setting or sector through the new project or service (e.g. providing a new or enhanced health service to the community) or gain new skills you could transfer to a completely different job – maybe leadership, project management, fundraising, research and enterprise skills.

Be clear about your rationale in writing the proposal and applying for funds before you prepare the financial budget for a bid. Understanding how much you or your organisation want to succeed in your bid will guide you as to the extent that you can undertake the proposed work at a loss to pump-prime a new field, or alternatively the minimum size of your profit margin. Factors to consider are:

- whether you have a reasonable chance of winning the bid. Rough out the costs of the time and resources of compiling the bid versus the likelihood of you being successful.
- why you want to make this bid. Initial losses could lead to future gains by establishing your track record in the field, and from associated contracts, succeeding in other linked bids on the basis of your newly established track record, and knowing more about future funding opportunities.
- whether your employing organisation requires you to make a surplus; this might be to meet organisational targets, finance equipment or key staff, fund research or maintain your department/area. Think whether your bid will be viable once these are factored in.
- what other bids/work you will lose out on whilst preparing or completing this bid, or actioning it if you are successful.
- if you already have the necessary resources to deliver (most of) the outcomes of the bid. These could be equipment, staff, skills, infrastructure, dissemination networks, time and money. Without these your bid may seem less competitive when compared with other agencies that are better endowed, unless your organisation will pump-prime basic resources with a view to attracting further commissions and establishing a high profile in the particular field in the future.
- whether your organisation is seen as 'suitable' to tender or operate the proposed project by the funding body. It is usual to submit details of your organisation's trading history, such as previous successful grants and current circumstances, to allow them to assess the level of risk of your successful delivery if you were to be awarded the bid.

To help you to decide whether to 'go' for a particular bid, review your previous success in attracting funds. Set up a spreadsheet with details of your bids over, say, the last three years. Ensure that you have calculated the full costs incurred in writing and preparing the bid, and add this, along with other relevant details such as the type of funding body, the value of the bid versus actual expenditure and outputs, etc. Use this exercise to review the various financial costs of bid preparation versus your success rates and in analysing other related factors and achievements. Discuss your tentative conclusions with colleagues or your line manager to get their perspectives too.

If, after this reality check, you are confident that it is worth the effort of going ahead with the bid, work through the five sections below to help you to prepare your budget.

Drawing up your budget

I How to work with your finance department

Involve your finance department as early as possible in preparing your application. Many organisations have rigorous financial procedures (and associated paperwork) to complete before an application for funding can be sent off. It will all be in vain if you have spent several weeks perfecting your application and networking with key players if you do not involve your finance department early on and your finance manager refuses to sign off your submission before the key deadline because of what they regard as unacceptable risks or weaknesses.

You or a suitable member of your bid team should be fully acquainted with the current finance procedures that need to be followed. Getting the timing right is essential; anticipate how long each step of the procedure takes. If the budget has to be approved by a committee, find out how often it meets and how long they need before the meeting to receive the necessary paperwork. Your finance team should consider the match between the overall proposed initiative, the draft budget and your organisation's strategic objectives. They will be familiar with the regulations that need to be fulfilled in parallel and the confirmatory signatures to be gained, before finance decisions can be taken. These might include research ethics approval and research governance agreement (see page 39), or other endorsements by the research and development lead of your organisation or department. The essential financial details likely to be required in the bid include:

- details of your organisation's bank account
- a copy of your organisation's indemnity insurance document
- detailed projected timesheets for staff working on the proposed project
- details of invoicing procedures and any prompt settlement discounts if these apply

- the name of the person responsible for your organisation's accounts.

There may also be standard costing forms that need to be completed and submitted to your organisation, different in format from those you have to include in the bid. For example a Transparent Approach to Costing (TRAC) has been accepted by the government, Funding Councils and Research Councils as 'an appropriate and robust method for costing in higher education'.[1,2] The costing methodology implemented by universities (Higher Education Institutions [HEIs]) based on TRAC costs is known as the calculation of full economic costs (fEC).

2 How to prepare your costings

Calculation of full economic costs is a requirement for HEIs. Your organisation may not be an HEI or required to use the TRAC method, and instead have its own standardised method, use historical data, calculate costings upon the basis of market demands, or negotiate over amounts. Even if you are not required to use fEC in your organisation, it does provide a useful basis for assessing the full costs involved in the proposed work. The suggestions for project costings described below reflect the fEC model. Indirect and estates cost rates have to be used when applying to the Research Councils for grants for research projects on a full economic cost basis and for projects awarded by other government departments.[1,2]

Staffing costs

Include the costs of staff directly employed to work on the project – for example, salaried staff in your organisation who will be employed solely or partly to work on this project for a fixed period of time. These costs should be directly calculable. There may be staff within your organisation who will provide input to the project and whose allocated time on the project needs to be estimated. This may include project leadership, administrative support, specialist or technical support, etc.

When calculating staff costs, use their full costs – which include any 'on-costs' such as the employer's contribution to the employee's pension and national insurance. Also take into account any incremental salary rises that will normally occur within the period of the project. Salaries should be indexed, that is linked to the estimated pay increases that will reflect inflation over the time period of the proposed project. Your finance or personnel departments should provide you with assistance for these calculations if necessary. They may have standard spreadsheets which you can utilise.

Expert advisors/contributors

You may plan to pay people to assist with the project who not directly employed by your organisation. These include advisors to contribute to or review the proposed work, independent consultants, casual staff, etc. Your finance and personnel departments should advise you about different payment or contractual methods, such as secondments, consultancy fees, honoraria, student bursaries, etc.

Calculating staff overheads

To fully cost the time of directly employed staff it is usual to add overheads to the project. This reflects the indirect and estate costs of employing the staff, such as upkeep of buildings, office space and equipment, central services departments (finance, personnel, library, catering, etc.) and general equipment not specified separately in the budget. This can be calculated in different ways and could be expressed as an added percentage to staffing costs. For example, prior to the introduction of fEC, some HEIs added between 46% and 103% to the total staff costs for research, consultancy or external work.

In HEIs, these indirect costs are now calculated separately, along with estate costs, according to the appropriate cost drivers.[1] The ways in which these costs are calculated differ between institutions, but total costs (not the rates for calculating them) must be shown if applying for research funding. If you are not required to use fEC, and your organisation does not have a fixed costing strategy, you may determine these overheads using national or market figures, or historical trading knowledge.

Additional expenses

Take into account all additional expenses, or you will be operating your proposed project at a loss and it will not be viable. There may be explicit information in the invitation to offer/bid for a project made by the funding body, regarding how additional expenses must be documented and how these can be claimed. Typical expenses you may directly incur include travel, overnight accommodation, venue hire, advertising, printing and postage. Include staff development/training in these costings, the expenses of presenting the findings at seminars and conferences, and any equipment you may require – such as laptops, desktop computers or technical aids.

Value Added Tax (VAT)

Include any applicable VAT in your projected costings. This will depend on whether your organisation is registered for VAT, or whether it has charitable status. Seek advice from your finance office about where VAT is payable, such as for secondments of project staff. VAT is generally non-recoverable by universities. It is important to ensure that any VAT that will be charged is included in your costings. The illustration provided in Table 5.1 indicates those items likely to incur VAT and those that generally will not. When preparing your costings, determine which costs include VAT (and check if your organisation is able to reclaim any VAT); then you can accurately reflect this in the project price. In the example in Table 5.1, external staff such as the external consultant authors will charge VAT (they are VAT registered) and this is therefore included in the costings.

Example

The costings outlined in Table 5.1 were for a development project at a university. the project was to create and pilot a toolkit to facilitate the involvement of patients in the teaching of health and social care students registered with the university. The costs include those arising from university staff directly employed to work on the project, and external consultant contributors (two authors contributed to writing and reviewing the toolkit; and a patient group was involved in teaching students, whose views were elicited in five focus groups). Expenses are included, such as the venue for the focus groups, refreshments, and travel expenses for patients. Additionally, staff travel and overnight expenses for the focus groups and meetings with contributing authors and the funding leads were incorporated. Costs for initial design and printing of the toolkit are included, although any additional costs for producing copies or hosting the toolkit as a downloadable document on a website are specifically excluded. Office expenses were included too: printer cartridges, stationery, photocopying, telephone expenses, postage, and any addi-

Table 5.1 Predicted costing for the development and piloting of a toolkit for involving patients in 'teaching and training' students

Staffing costs for twelve-month period in one tax year		VAT
Directly employed staff (costs based on Full Time Equivalent (FTE) staff time, including 'on-costs' i.e. employer's contributions to pension and national insurance payments for the employee)		
Project lead	0.4 FTE	£18,721 n/a
Project officer	Full time (1 FTE)	£24,500 n/a
Project assistant	0.6 FTE	£10,800 n/a
Sub-total of staffing FTEs	2.0 FTE	
Overhead rate calculated per FTE	£35,000 per research FTE (NB varies per institution)	£70,000 n/a
External consultant contributors		
Expert consultant authors	2 @ £350 per day for 5 days each inc. VAT	£2,979 £521
Patient contributors	9 x 2-hour focus groups; up to 10 patients @ £8 each per hour	£1,440 n/a
Non-staff expenses		
Refreshments for 9 focus groups inc VAT		£64 £11
Staff travel and overnight accommodation inc VAT		£1,702 £298
Patient group travel expenses		£500 n/a
Venue hire for focus groups inc VAT		£851 £149
Print and design of toolkits (80 @ £16.50 + VAT each)		£1,320 £231
Library expenses		£60 n/a
Office expenses inc VAT		£2,723 £477
Staff development, conferences, training inc VAT		£1,277 £223
Sub-total non-staff expenses		£8,497 £1,389
		Total cost £13,8847

tional office equipment necessary to complete the project such as recording devices for the focus group discussions and transcribing equipment. Staff development included training courses and back-fill expenses. Conferences and meetings necessary for staff to complete this work or disseminate the findings should also be included.

Staffing costs (as shown in Table 5.1) are calculated using the annual salary of the staff member plus the pension and national insurance contributions which the organisation has to pay for the staff member, termed the 'on-costs'. These costs vary according to an individual's salary level (your organisation's human resources or payroll department will furnish details). Calculate the FTE rate for the staff member by working out the length of time spent on the project as a proportion of the annual number of hours worked (for a university researcher, typically 1650 hours). For example, if the annual salary of the project lead is £38,343 and the organisation's additional pension and national insurance contributions ('on-costs') are £8,460, the total of £46,803 would be equivalent to 1650 hours or 1.0 FTE. So if the period of time spent on the project was approximately full-time for four months – or the equivalent of two days a week for one year – this would be 660 hours or 0.4 FTE and would be shown as a cost of £18,721.

Costing strategy

Your next step is to set the price. To a certain extent this will depend on the type of contract for which you are bidding. For some bids the final cost is fixed and includes all your expenses and any VAT. However, other commissioners may expect you to claim separately for certain expenses, so read all of the information in the invitation to bid.

The strategy you employ to reach the final total may depend on your organisation's needs and aspirations, knowledge of your competitors' likely bids, or knowledge of the funding body's target price for the project. The upper limit of the price of the project may be set out in the notes of the invitation to bid, and you will then need to identify, using a full costing method, whether your organisation can complete the project for this price limit.

3. How to plan for additional expenses

It is difficult to plan for every eventuality in your costings, particularly if a project is running over a considerable period of time. Staff may leave, go off on long-term sickness leave, or fail to fulfil the project requirements. You will incur additional costs for these eventualities. Negotiation with the funding body for additional money in the future may be a possibility, but this is not likely.

You must decide on your contingency plans. You could build additional sums into the project costing, such as staff development money, that might be diverted to a different purpose by agreement if that became necessary. In the event that additional expenses are not needed, this sum could then be used for its original purpose at the end of the project, such as giving conference presentations about the completed project and its outputs. Or your untouched contingency funds could provide resources for pump-priming another initiative, or for a team-building event to share good practice and plan for future funding opportunities, or for achieving organisational and/or personal objectives.

4. How to present your budget in the bid

The budget in your final bid submission may differ in format from the costings required by your organisation. For example, many organisations will expect you to complete a particular table/spreadsheet so that they can easily compare one proposed budget with another. To submit complex forms such as those required for costing a possible project by your organisation may be detrimental to you winning the bid.

With any bid, and particularly with complex ones, it is likely that many revisions will be made before submission of the final copy. Additionally there may be a large number of people in your bidding team at any one time reviewing and revising the material. This increases the likelihood of errors going unnoticed in the final submission. Costing errors are easily made as any changes to the scope or content of the bid are likely to result in the budget being recalculated. See Box 5.1 for tips on how to minimise errors in costing a bid.

It is vital to check and re-check any figures you present in the bid. Any mistakes could be very costly for your organisation if an offer

---

Box 5.1 Top tips to minimise errors in costing a bid

- Have a system for numbering or dating draft versions, e.g. including the version number in the page footer
- Use colour when you make changes so that they are easy to spot
- Give one team member the responsibility for amending the budget to match any revisions in the content of the proposal
- Allow dedicated time, prior to submitting the final version of the bid, to systematically check the entire submission including the budget. This task should ideally be performed by the senior person with lead responsibility for making the bid
- Do not forget to include VAT where applicable.

is accepted on the basis of erroneous figures which are too low. An otherwise good bid will be judged harshly if the evaluators think that errors in calculations indicate inefficiency in the bidding team.

Illustrative example bid

The following tables illustrate methods of presentation that you may choose to use when preparing your budget. The costings in Tables 5.2, 5.3, 5.4 and 5.5 all relate to the provision and delivery of a training programme in communication skills. Costs are based on the initial set up, design and pilot of the programme. The upper limit of the bid price has been set at £60,000.

Table 5.2 illustrates how the total costs for staff time on the project are calculated.

Table 5.2 Example costings of staff input in the development and delivery of training programme

Employed staff	Number of hours (estimated)	Rate/hour (inclusive of 'on-costs', VAT and overheads)	Total cost
Project lead (PL)	160	£55	£8,800
Senior trainer/lecturer (SL)	420	£40	£16,800
Course facilitator (CF)	80	£35	£2,800
Project Manager (PM)	360	£35	£12,600
Technical support (TS)	50	£30	£1,500
Administrative support (AS)	300	£25	£7,500
Expert contributors (EC)	90	£40	£3,600
Total estimated hours	**1460**		
Average hourly rate		**£36.71**	
Total staff costs			**£53,600**

Using the figures in Table 5.2 you can produce another spreadsheet indicating how the work for each part of the project is broken down. This could include the staff involved in each part of the project and their estimated hours which would then provide a costing for each component of the project, as shown in Table 5.3. Project expenses should also be given and added to staff costings to give a total project price as in Table 5.4.

Table 5.3 Extent and associated costs of staff input in each component of the training programme

Project component	Staff member	Hours (estimated number for each staff member respectively)	Hourly rate (£) (inc. 'on-costs', VAT and over-heads where applicable for each staff member respectively)	Cost of each component of project (£)
Project set up/ preliminary work	PL, SL, PM	30, 40, 30	55, 40, 35	4,300
Design of the programme	PL, SL, PM, EC, CF, AS	45, 130, 70, 30, 20, 103	55, 40, 35, 40, 35, 25	14,600
Accreditation of the programme	PL, SL, PM, EC, CF, AS	30, 50, 40, 20, 10, 30	55, 40, 35, 40, 35, 25	6,950
Preparation of web-based support	PM, TS	20, 50	35, 30	2,200
Delivery of core workshops	SL, PM, AS	150, 130, 120	40, 35, 25	13,550
Delivery of additional action learning sets – facilitated in participants' workplaces	CF, PM, EC	50, 45, 20	35, 35, 40	4,125
Evaluation of programme	PL, SL, PM, EC, AS	45, 40, 20, 20, 37	55, 40, 35, 40, 25	6,500
Preparation of final reports	PL, SL, PM, AS	10, 10, 5, 10	55, 40, 35, 25	1,375
Total staff costs				**53,600**

Table 5.4 Total budget for training programme including staff and non-staff costs

Total budget	
Sub-total cost for staff time	£53,600
Sub-total costs for travel and accommodation	£ 2,300
Sub-total costs for office expenses (post, telephone, office space and equipment, photocopying, printing, etc.)	£ 3,800
Sub-total costs of venue, refreshments	£ 280
Total project price	**£59,980**

An alternative approach to summarising your budget is shown in Table 5.5. This indicates the predicted costing for each component of the project. This can be a particularly useful method if you need to negotiate the inclusion of specific project components with the funding body. The approach can also be used to agree a payment schedule with your funding body, with set payments and dates given for each component of the project.

5. Plan how to respond to questions about the budget from the interview panel once you are shortlisted

It is best if the person with financial responsibility can join the bidding team to face the panel if you are interviewed; but if not, it is essential that one of the bidding team assumes responsibility for answering budgetary questions. These may include questions relating to:

- *Negotiable aspects of the project.* If possible decide for which, if any, parts of the project proposal you are prepared to negotiate the price, with additional costs or deductions in proportion to adding in, scaling down or omitting certain components of the project. If you are questioned on costings for additional services or deductions that you had not prepared for, agree to consider this and take time to give new costings after the interview. Avoid making a quick decision to secure the bid and then finding that, when new costings are prepared, you are working at a loss.
- *Value added tax (VAT).* There may be questions on clarification relating to the inclusion or exclusion of VAT on some or all parts of the project budget. Which expenses do and do not incur VAT will depend on the status of your organisation, the nature of any

Table 5.5 Project budget representing costings per individual tasks/components

Project component	Project timetable	Total estimated cost per component (£) (including 'on costs', VAT and overheads where applicable)
Project set up/preliminary work Initial meeting, confirm project outline, contact key stakeholders and contributors, etc.	Jan–March	5,000
Design of the programme	March–June	15,600
Accreditation of the programme*	May–July	7,400
Preparation of web based support	April–July	2,200
Delivery of core workshops	August–October	14,900
Delivery of additional action learning sets – facilitated in participants' workplaces	Sept–November	5,380
Evaluation of the programme*	Aug–December	8,000
Preparation of final reports		1,500
Total project price		**59,980**

*These components could be project tasks that are rated as desirable, rather than essential, and give 'added value'; you may wish to negotiate pricing based on their inclusion or exclusion from the project. You may prefer to illustrate this by showing comparative budgets with and without these components in separate tables. You could also consider providing a tiered approach to pricing, for example by giving illustrative budgets varying from basic prices for a low-level evaluation to a more costly and more complex model; or in-house accreditation to a national approach taken by a university.

consultant contributors and the type of expenses, so seek specific advice from your finance department.

- *How costs will be recorded.* It may be that there are specific requirements for keeping records of payments, staff time sheets, etc. These can vary but are generally provided in detail by the fund holder. (If details are not provided in the initial documentation from the funding body, look on their website, and, if this does not help, your finance department may be an invaluable source of advice.)

How to manage your budget

Once the project is running you must ensure that the budget is managed efficiently to keep within your set costings. Some good tips on managing your budget are:

- Keep accurate records of your expenditure (including details such as staff timesheets, records of telephone calls, etc., if these are required by the funding body).
- Review the budget monthly using your financial reports (ensure you know how to obtain reports from your finance team and how your budget reports should be recorded).
- Retain and file all necessary finance documentation, including receipts and claims for income/expenditure, etc.
- Know how long you need to keep all necessary documentation. This includes the period of time required by both your organisation and the funding body for audit purposes. If you cannot justify your income and expenditure with appropriate documentation then your organisation may have to repay some or all of the project funds.

Be clear about the final price you have agreed with the funding provider. Is this a set price provided that you deliver the minimum agreed services or exceed these services? What will happen if these costs are under or over budget? If you go over budget it is likely that your organisation will have to cover these extra costs unless this was previously specifically agreed with the funding body and written confirmation is obtained. You will need to manage this either by budgeting to recover these additional costs in another part of the project (whilst maintaining quality and delivery of the project component) or by agreeing the budget overspend with your project lead/finance department, for instance by reducing your projected surplus. If you deliver the project under budget and have a surplus of money you had not expected, you need to determine if this should be repaid to the funding provider. This may not be necessary or appropriate if the specified project work has been completed satisfactorily to at least the minimum expectations and within the proposed time frame. You can check this with the funding body's conditions of offer or, if this is unclear, with your finance department. If you do have surplus finances that are retained by your organisation at the end of a project, it is good if you can agree to reinvest these funds to pump-prime another pilot project or to plan or draw up a future bid. Consider if the surplus funds could be used to mainstream the project or take it forward? You could use the funds to expand your team, or to buy essential equipment to help support future funding applications.

Final tips on preparing the proposed budget for your bid

1 Think of the various sources of funding and current resources relevant to your proposed project. Don't consider the budget you draw up for the bid in isolation. There will be other resources in your organisation, or within your other allied or current projects, or in the collaborating organisations for your bid. The more 'free goods' that you include, or potential additional resources, the more 'value for money' the funding body will perceive within your budget and the more realistic they will rate your chances of completing the contract.

2 Determine the normal overhead charges by the organisation hosting the bid and the collaborating organisations at the outset. If you think that the overheads are too high and will limit what work you can offer in your bid, or that they will mean you can only afford junior rather than senior staffing, see if you can negotiate a lower overhead in some way. Maybe you can convince your organisation that it should invest to 'pump-prime' your work in the field, to enhance the organisation's profile or to feed into another of its divisions to create new business opportunities (e.g. to enhance teaching). Another option might be to see if another collaborating organisation has lower overheads and could host the budget with a lower budgetary charge overall. Or persuade the organisation(s) charging greater than 100% overhead charges to include a mass of resources within this overhead 'tax', such as secretarial and administration staff, office expenses, travel, library, premises, recruitment costs, etc.

3 Consider salary costs, and how these will increase with inflation and increasing tenure in the post in successive years if the proposed project spans several years; if the project starts in the next financial year, don't forget to price the salaries at next year's rates.

4 If you are a novice at drawing up and managing a budget, then seek and obtain expert help throughout the process, even if you feel you are being a nuisance with your continual questioning.

References

1 Joint Costing and Pricing Steering Group, Higher Education Funding Council for England (HEFCE). *Transparent approach to costing: An overview of TRAC.* Bristol: HEFCE; 2005.

2 www.hefce.ac.uk/finance/fundinghe/TransparencyReview

Chapter 6

Succeeding at the interview

Ruth Chambers

Some funding bodies allocate awards without a face-to-face interview, but substantial awards almost invariably progress, through shortlisting outline applications, to development of applications, then further shortlisting of full applications, and to personal interviews of the bidding teams by panels of experts appointed by the funding body.

Preparing for the interview

Once shortlisted you should capitalise on your resources and past achievements. Use the presentation on a given topic or your full bid to give a slick demonstration of your communication, organisational and information technology skills, as well as the content of the proposal itself.

Find out who is on the interview panel by ringing the contact person given in the letter inviting you for interview, assuming that the letter does not include the information. If you know who is on the panel and the posts they hold, you will be better able to prepare for the type and content of questions they will pose at interview.

Obtain a copy of the annual report of the funding body. It will help you to gauge the size and strength of their organisation, as well as give you information on which to base intelligent questions or describe your plans, to match the organisation's priorities and values.

Decide how much you want the work, and what compromises you can make in what you are offering to provide for the amount of money or resources on offer.

Do not assume that all those on the interview panel can remember the details of your proposal or your CVs – or have even read them thoroughly. Emphasise your strengths and experience as you give your presentation or reply to their questions.

Prepare a short aide-memoire or handout that you can leave behind, so that they can remember you easily. Nothing too ostentatious though. Ascertain what audiovisual equipment will be available for presentation, and what you need to bring yourself. If you use Microsoft's PowerPoint for your presentation your hand-out should include a copy (in colour) for each panel member as well as a copy of any other achievements or substantiating information you want them to note. Take along visually attractive work that shows you have succeeded in previous commissions, e.g. toolkits, publications, interactive tools, inventions.

Anticipate the interview questions as far you are able; and prepare answers. Field a project team that will be able to answer questions from the panel and demonstrate the richness and diversity of the team or their special attributes and reliability. Choreograph your performance. You all need to appear credible to all the members of the interview panel, whatever your individual roles in the overall project.

Consider beforehand if there is any part of the proposal that you could negotiate on if asked at interview – such as content, scope, costings, etc.

The big day

Dress to impress. Old fashioned advice? You are trying to sell yourself as competent, capable and credible.

By the time you are called for an interview, the panel have already seen much in your application that makes them want to consider awarding funding to you. Remember this, if you are starting to flounder, and regain your positive mental attitude.

The panel's first few questions should be designed to put you at your ease and settle your nerves. Make eye contact, smile and look interested. Try to remember the names of people on the panel; make a quick note of their names and posts as they are introduced to you if you can do so whilst retaining eye contact. Avoid responding "It is all there in our application form" to a question from the panel. This is your opportunity to describe your work, hopes and values.

Do not antagonise interview panels by automatically questioning or arguing a point unless you can do so in a considered way. But if you basically disagree with the panel representing the funding body, consider how you will work with an organisation that does not think in a similar way to you. The interview may be the first time that you realise that you and your potential source of funding are incompatible. Be honest with yourself and the interview panel.

Some questions can be unnerving if you do not know the answer. The best thing is to admit your ignorance but say how you would go about finding out.

Find the balance between thinking before you speak and thinking out loud if you are unsure about an answer. Interviewers may be interested in how you approach a question even if you do not know instantly what they are driving at. If you do put your foot in it, do not dig any deeper. It should be okay to say "Actually, now I think about it, that's a daft answer", and have another go at it. Or ask them to rephrase the question for you (but only do that once in the interview).

Honesty and integrity show through. Do not try to second guess the 'correct' answer. Politics may be discussed. Say what you think and try to justify it.

Tips on succeeding at the interview[1]

- Field presenters with diverse experience that cover the remit of the tender as far as possible.
- If there is a 'gap' in your presenting team, talk to experts relevant to your 'gap' so you can confidently address related questions from the interview panel.
- Dress smartly – all of you; if there is a lot of money and potential up for grabs, informal dress can indicate a casual approach in the eyes of the panel.
- Initiate eye contact with all members of the panel, but particularly the person asking the question.
- Keep your presentation to time; clarify the time allowed before you start if it is not specified by the panel chair, in case it differs from the briefing notes.
- Introduce everyone on the presenting team before you start, and before the allotted time for the presentation.
- Do not be put off by being kept waiting for your allotted slot.
- Ask if you can arrange for your presentation to be loaded onto the computer before your interview; and check that the panel assumes responsibility for the technical side.
- Produce handouts, copying your presentation (if using Power-Point) or summarising key points (if not using audiovisual equipment); decide if it is best to give material out at the start of the interview, at the end of the presentation, or just before you leave the interview. Consider whether it is best to provide space for notes on each page, handouts in colour, a logo or other iden-

tifier on each page, and handouts in the official folder or presentation pack.

• Consider how to provide evidence of your profile or relevant achievement which you can leave behind, e.g. reports or similar documents you have produced, or other outputs of initiatives you have conducted.

• Read and re-read the tender or bid document and any associated background papers relating to the purpose of the project or service(s) covered by the tender or bid, including the values and beliefs of the funding organisation. Pitch your presentation at these, and craft your content and style to match the nature of the tender or bid, and of the funding organisation.

• Agree who will deliver the presentation and who will respond to the range of questions you expect the panel to pose. Beware of having more than one presenter to give a 10–15 minute presentation in case it appears fragmented or in danger of over-running the allotted time.

• As in any interview, think through what questions you wish to ask the panel so that you are fully aware of what the 'job' or commission would entail. Any substantial questions or reservations should have been cleared up before getting as far as the presentation. But things change, and there may have been recent developments that impact on your tender or the viability of the project. Confine yourself to one or at most two questions for the panel (if invited to pose questions) that may have arisen as a result of the interview and discussion that has just taken place. This will emphasise your insightful perspectives and quick thinking.

• Say hello and smile as you enter the room and take your place, whether or not you know the panel members; establish rapport.

• Look at the visitors' register on the front desk as you sign in on your arrival; who are your competitors; what advantage do you have over them that you can plug at the interview?

• Portray your team as a no-risk option.

Dealing with the questions and discussion[2]

Demonstrate your skills in inviting and answering questions following on from your presentation by:

• *Exuding self confidence:* establish good eye contact, smiling appropriately

• *Your honesty:* answer questions honestly. If you don't know, say so. Do prepare answers to questions you can anticipate being almost sure you'll get

- *Eliminating nervous habits:* fiddling with your rings and playing with your hair are out
- *Making the most of your visual material*
- *Keeping your discussion simple and to the point:* avoid jargon and technical words unless you plan to use those purposely to illustrate how in tune you are with the funding body
- *Referring to sources of evidence:* use these to justify your answers if that is appropriate
- *Expressing gratitude:* thank the panel before you close for the time given and interest shown.

Making an effective PowerPoint presentation

Your presentation should be well structured, with at least an introduction, a main body and a conclusion. Look at Box 6.1 for a reminder about how to give an effective presentation. It will be challenging and a bit of a performance, as a great deal depends on your presentation and the way the panel interpret your bid. It's the culmination of weeks or months of work, preparing and submitting your bid. Nevertheless you need to give out an aura of confidence and being at ease, making a concerted effort to engage the panel members and hold their interest. You can find out more about designing and organising your presentation at <u>funsan.biomed. mcgill.ca/~funnell/InforMed/Bacon/Present/pres.html</u>.

Box 6.1 Giving an effective PowerPoint presentation[3]

- Choose a format for your presentation that is in keeping with the theme of your talk.
- Use clear, legible text in short phrases or sentences.
- Match the font size to the size of the room: e.g. use 24pt characters in a typical interview room.
- Include only one idea per screen.
- Limit yourself to six or less words per line, and six or less lines.
- Predominantly lower-case letters are more easy to read than CAPITALS.
- Maximise the contrast between text and background.
- Build your PowerPoint slides into a logical sequence for the presentation.
- Stay calm, and use a printout of your slides as handouts, if the PowerPoint equipment is not working on the day.

References

1   Jay R. *Effective Presentation*. The Institute of Management Foundation. London: Pitman Publishing; 1995.

2   Kiani F. Post-presentation questions. *BMJcareers*. 2006; 8 April : gp137.

3   Holzl J. Twelve tips for effective PowerPoint presentations for the technologically challenged. *Medical Teacher*. 1997. **19**: 175-9.

Chapter 7

Understanding the funding body's perspective

Ruth Chambers

You will be more likely to be successful in making a bid if you pitch your bid so that is as near as possible to what the funding body is asking for. To do that you need to understand the purpose and aim of the bid as it is described in any documentation supplied by the funding body. This chapter should help you to consider the funding body's perspective – the context of the award, their values and beliefs, and their reasons for offering the funding in the first place. The more you appreciate their perspective, the better you can prepare your proposal to match their requirements and preferences.

Some insights into funding research

Funding bodies may be local, regional, national or international in scope. They fund research in two basic ways – by way of either:

- a contract to undertake a specific piece of research that is requested by the funding body; or
- an open competition in a field of research for which the funding body has a specific remit.[1]

Those judging your bid should understand what constitutes high-quality research or the equivalent if funding other types of posts, projects or service developments. They should be familiar with the type of methodology that is most likely to answer the purpose they have expressed in their award details. Different types of question will require different kinds of evidence to answer them. In each case the assessors will rate the risks that a chosen methodology or particular bidding organisation can provide irrefutable evidence to answer that question.

Assume that the shortlisting criteria are derived from the purpose, aims and objectives of the invitation to bid or to tender, the expected outcomes, the nature of the target population at whom the 'project' is aimed, if these are not given in the funding body's invitation.

The funding body may consider that the hierarchy of evidence, as given in Box 7.1, reflects the likelihood that the evidence gained by those conducting a study will result in certain knowledge. Obviously the funding body will hope that the work they pay for leads to clear evidence that the intervention being researched, or the new service being set up, is beneficial (see Box 7.2).

Once the funding body has established that your research application is within their remit, it will pose four questions:[2]

1 Is this an important research question?
2 Should we support a study that seeks to answer this question?
3 Will this particular study answer this question?
4 Do these investigators have the skills, resources and support from others to bring this study to a successful conclusion?

So there will be many factors to take into account when a funding body is gauging the quality of a bid, as was illustrated by the case study in Chapter 4. These factors include establishing that:[3]

- the ethos of the individual or organisation bidding suits that of the funding body and purpose of the award
- the nature of the proposed design is fit for purpose
- the size of the study is feasible and valid as to number of subjects, area covered, extent of the intervention, etc.
- the proposed type of study is relevant to the purpose
- the track record of the bidding individual or organisation is sufficient: do they usually do what they promise, are they efficient and effective, what sort of publicity do they usually generate from their work, are they ethical?
- the extent of preliminary work already undertaken will contribute to the overall study
- the predicted timescale is realistic
- the extent of resources said to be being contributed by the bidding individual or organisation exists
- the extent of resources requested is sufficient to fulfil the purpose and aim of the commission
- the tools proposed to be used in the method or interpretation of the results are valid and reliable
- the way that the proposed project is conducted – in other words the proposed recruitment and selection of subjects, drop out rates, length and type of follow-up – will be of high quality
- the statistical methods proposed – for example the power of the results as derived from the size of the proposed study, confi-

---

Box 7.1 Strength of evidence[4]

Type I: Strong evidence from at least one systematic review of multiple well-designed randomised controlled trials (RCTs).

Type II   Strong evidence from at least one properly designed randomised controlled trial of appropriate size.

Type III   Evidence from well-designed trials without randomisation, single group pre-post, cohort, time series or matched case-control studies.

Type IV   Evidence from well-designed non-experimental studies from more than one centre or research group.

Type V   Opinions of respected authorities, based on clinical evidence, descriptive studies or reports of expert committees.

---

dence intervals around the point estimates of the effects of the study – will enable valid conclusions to be made.

See Box 7.1 for a classification that is often used to grade the strength of evidence.

Another way of categorising evidence is described in the compendium *Clinical Evidence*, which is updated every six months. This perspective of evidence can be applied by health professionals in their everyday work; see Box 7.2.[5]

Box 7.2 Evidence of benefits

Beneficial: Interventions whose effectiveness has been shown by clear evidence from controlled trials.

Likely to be beneficial: Interventions for which effectiveness is less well established than for those listed under 'beneficial'.

Trade-off between benefits and harms: Interventions for which clinicians and patients should weigh up the beneficial and harmful effects according to individual circumstances and priorities.

Unknown effectiveness: Interventions for which there are currently insufficient data or data of inadequate quality (includes interventions that are widely accepted as beneficial but have never been formally tested in RCTs, often because RCTs would be regarded as unethical).

Unlikely to be beneficial: Interventions for which the lack of effectiveness is less well established than for those listed under 'likely to be ineffective or harmful'.

Likely to be ineffective or harmful: Interventions whose ineffectiveness or harmfulness have been demonstrated by clear evidence.

Why proposals are rejected

There may be reasons why the potential funding that is advertised is later withdrawn so that all the proposals received are therefore discarded. There may be a range of political, business, budgetary or personal reasons why funding is withdrawn. For instance, if the funding body merges with one or more other organisations, or is taken over by an umbrella organisation with a different ethos or vision, then new or current funding awards may be frozen until it has established its priorities or work programme. Even if funding is reinstated at a later date, circumstances will have changed, requiring you to rethink your proposal to ensure that it is still relevant.

Box 7.3 relays a range of reasons why research proposals are rejected. These reasons can be generalised to all types of proposals, so make sure that you do not fall into any of these potential traps.

Essentially you must adhere to the funding body's specifications and preferences. These will include[6] their:

- Priorities – in general and specific to the bid
- Inclusions in relation to resources contributed
- Exclusions – what they will and will not fund
- Expectations in relation to co-funding by your organisation or by your partners
- Attitude to intellectual property
- Ethical and political standpoints
- Application format and process
- Assessment process and criteria for the various stages (e.g. outline application and full application, as described in Chapter 4)
- Deadlines.

The tendering procedure

The organisation offering the funding will have standard contract conditions under which they work. They will compile, or procure from another body or organisation, lists of approved organisations and individuals from whom tenders and quotations may be invited. Individuals or organisations may apply for permission to tender or quote for future work, such as the supply of goods, materials, training, project or consultancy services, and the commissioning organisation will have a system to rate their technical and professional competence and financial standing.

Sometimes there is no list of approved firms or individuals in cases where specialist services or skills are required, or there are

Box 7.3 Why proposals are rejected[7]

Problem addressed

- Not of sufficient importance
- Proposal not likely to produce sufficiently new or useful information
- Proposed research based on insufficient evidence
- Proposed method is unsound
- Problem is more complex than the investigator appears to realise
- Problem addressed or research proposed is too local; needs to be able to be generalised
- It would be more appropriate to undertake a pilot study than a full-blown research project
- The proposal is too complicated and involves too many elements to be explored simultaneously
- The proposal is vague without a specific aim.

Approach proposed

- The scope or type of the method is not suitable for the aim or purpose of the commission
- There is not enough detail about the methods proposed
- The overall design of the project proposed has not been clearly thought out
- The statistics underpinning the proposed work have not been considered in sufficient detail
- Equipment proposed is not suitable or up to date.

Investigators proposed

- Appear to be unfamiliar with the published literature, the field, current thinking or methodology
- Track records do not inspire confidence
- Insufficient experience and capacity in proposed team
- Proposed investigators appear isolated from key people in the field; they have too few collaborators.

Other

- Lack of trust in organisation proposing to undertake the commission
- Competing commitments and pressures on proposed investigators or their organisation may distract them from concentrating on the proposed work
- Current research grants or other funding attracted are already adequate to undertake the proposed work.

insufficient suitable potential contractors on the approved list. Then the technical and financial capability of organisations invited to tender or quote will be scrutinised specifically as part of the tendering process.

The commissioning organisation will be looking for 'value for money' and to see whether the number of tenders received provides adequate competition. If there are too few, it may be that individuals or organisations who could undertake the work more cheaply or productively have not submitted a bid or were not invited to tender, in which case the invitation to tender should be widened before a decision about awarding the tender is made. There would have to be good reasons not to accept the lowest tender; the commissioning organisation will have to weigh the actual or potential benefits and risks associated with a more costly proposal compared with the lowest tender.

Formal tendering procedures may be waived by senior people in the commissioning organisation if the estimated finance involved is expected to be within certain financial limits; see Box 1.3 for an example. Other reasons why a commissioning organisation would not employ a formal tendering process include:[8]

*   their umbrella organisation instructs them to comply with its special arrangements with a provider
*   the timescale is so urgent it genuinely precludes competitive tendering
*   the specialist expertise required is only available from one source, so there is no possibility of setting up a tendering process (as long as the commissioning organisation has genuinely tried to seek out such specialists)
*   the new work is really a continuation of previous work and it makes sense to re-appoint the previous consultants or organisation to undertake the new task. The benefits of such continuity must outweigh any potential financial advantage to be gained by competitive tendering.

Selection of panel members for shortlisting and interviewing

The funding body will probably have tried to recruit a wide spread of key stakeholders to shortlist the submissions and make up the interview panel, so consider their perspectives in finalising your submission and preparing for the interview (see Chapter 6).

Peer review

A funding body may include peer review of individual proposals or bids in their grant awarding process. Sometimes those submitting a bid name a range of people who would be prepared to peer-review the proposal if invited to do so by the sponsor, although the peer reviewers actually chosen may not be taken from the range. As many as six people might read your application (in confidence), and score it or comment on the quality and feasibility of the proposal (see Table 4.1 for an example): that the proposed project has a reasonable chance of being completed in the predicted time frame according to the protocol.[1] Sometimes the issues raised as concerns or suggestions by the referees are fed back to the applicants to give them a chance to address the issues in their full application or at interview, as was described in the case study in Chapter 4.

Peer review has been criticised for its lack of objectivity or reliability (as summed up by Smith in Box 7.4[9]). It is a subjective and inconsistent process dependent on the perspectives of the chosen reviewers and the knowledge and attitudes of the individual chairing the funding body's award committee.

Box 7.4 Reviewing peer review[9]

But who is a peer? Somebody doing exactly the same kind of research (in which case he or she is probably a direct competitor)? Somebody in the same discipline? Somebody who is an expert on methodology? And what is review? Somebody saying 'The paper looks alright to me'...Or somebody poring all over the paper, asking for raw data, repeating analyses, checking all the references, and making detailed suggestions for improvements? Such a review is vanishingly rare.

References

1 Brown N. *What a funder looks for*. In: The Times Higher Education. *How to get a research grant. A guide for academics*, The Times Higher Education Supplement; 2005.

2 Usherwood T. *Introduction to project management in health research. A guide for new researchers*. Buckingham: Open University Press; 1996.

3 Glasziou P, Vandenbroucke J, Chalmers I. Assessing the quality of research. *BMJ*. 2004; 328: 39–41.

4 Muir Gray JA. *Evidence-based Healthcare*. Edinburgh: Churchill Livingstone; 1997.

5 Tovey D (editor). *Clinical Evidence*. Issue 14. London: BMJ Publishing Group; 2005.

6 Kenway J, Boden R, Epstein D. *Winning and managing research funding.* London: SAGE; 2005.

7 Allen EM. Why proposals are rejected. *Science.* 1960; 132: 1532–4.

8 Hampshire & Isle of Wight Strategic Health Authority. *Corporate Governance Manual.* Hampshire: Hampshire & Isle of Wight SHA; 2003.

9 Smith R. Peer review: a flawed process at the heart of science and journals. *J R Soc Med.* 2006; 99: 178–82.

Chapter 8

Writing a bid from a novice's perspective

Anne Longbottom and Sara Buckley

This chapter is written by two project managers new to research and project programmes. It gives their personal experiences of learning about writing bids and putting the funded projects into action.

Where do you start?

As someone new to writing bids it can all seem a little daunting. However, everyone has to start somewhere. One of the most important things to consider is to think about whom you could invite to be involved in submitting a bid with you, and what skills and knowledge you and they could bring to a potential project.

We were fortunate that we had a project leader who was experienced in writing bids and had previously undertaken numerous projects for a variety of different organisations. So she understood what would be expected from all of us in her project team if we were to be successful. This gave us the opportunity as project managers to develop the projects for which we gained funding, under her expert guidance, in the knowledge that we had good support whenever it was needed.

Reputation is very important. We were told at a workshop, 'You are only as good as the last job you [as an individual; as an organisation] have done.' Each bid has to be written as if it is the most special application for funding you have made. Getting others' perspectives can help you to focus on what is important.

Box 8.1 on page 104 gives some tips for beginners to research as they begin to make their first bids.

Box 8.1 Research for beginners[1]

Focus on these priorities:

- Research is always more complicated than it initially seems. Beginners grossly underestimate the practical difficulties and time needed for each stage of the project.
- Choose your supervisor carefully. If you have a choice, undertake your research under the guidance of an experienced supervisor (you can see how important this is from the case studies presented in this chapter). Keep your supervisor updated, and share problems early.
- Read the study proposal again and again. Make sure you understand it and appreciate the meaning of the aims and objectives.
- Secure the necessary approvals in good time: from your trust, university, research ethics committees, NHS Caldicott Guardian, laboratory or other organisation.
- Set up your database properly.
- Be organised. This means anticipating resources in setting up the study, practising good time management, writing up your work as you go along, reviewing newly published literature.
- Maintain good working relationships with everyone involved in the research study.

Enthusiasm versus realism

Proposals and bids may take weeks, even months, to put together, so you need to be realistic about what you bid for and whom you include in the process to help you. Building a good team around you is very important to the success of the project; you need to understand each individual's strengths and weaknesses, their potential and what they can contribute. The team's knowledge and skills are central resources to the bid you are writing. Even if you intend to work alone on a project, you will still need support from other people – for example, as critical friends.

People may be flattered if they're asked to take part in a project, and they may get carried away with ideas and promise more of their time than they can actually afford. The time between writing the outline bid and actually achieving funding can be considerable – maybe as much as a year – and the people that you expected to be involved in your project may by then have taken on other roles, or be fully employed elsewhere, as their circumstances have changed over time.

Case study A

(Anne Longbottom)

I was approached to join a team which was putting together a bid to develop an electronic toolkit as part of a larger project to facilitate the employment, recruitment and retention of health-care assistants in general practice. The bid was submitted, and my role was to present the tender to the commissioners of the toolkit. At the time I was working within the NHS to coordinate, and increase the level of access to, training for non-professionally-qualified staff within seven NHS trusts in the local area.

When I first saw the project proposal I was surprised to see how involved it was. It described the rationale for why the proposal had been submitted, the people who supported the bid and what the final product might look. It included detailed financial information about how any money received would be spent. The most complicated part of the bid described the different levels of work that could be expected for varying levels of finance. There were staggered bids at three levels, and each component of the bid added a unique piece to the 'jigsaw'. The aim was to produce the best possible product at each costing level, but to make the next level seem too good an opportunity for the commissioners to miss. All the time it was important to bear in mind our capabilities and limitations as a small project team.

It took around three months from our first expression of interest in submitting a tender to being shortlisted and going to interview. It then took another two months before the final contracts were agreed and work could start.

Be aware of sources of funding

Details of projects for which funding is available, and invitations for expressions of interest, may be posted on websites or in journals long before the full bidding details are available, and it can be hard work keeping track of all that is on offer. There are websites dedicated to different areas of expertise. For example, a researcher or member of staff working in a subscribing organisation can register for the UKRO information services at the UK Research Office website, ims.ukro.ac.uk. This can deliver information tailored to your own specific research and policy interests. See page 12 for information about other sources of funding.

Some funding bodies give full details of what they expect the project to achieve, and your job is to tell them how you can fulfil their needs. Other funding bodies are looking for new ideas and offer support for innovative projects.

Networking is a good way of finding out what funding is available. Let people know your areas of interest or expertise and they may suggest funding opportunities as they arise. Our project leader regularly attends national meetings, and often finds out about as yet unadvertised funding opportunities there.

Within the university we have an external projects team employed to gather information about sources of funding and their funding criteria. They maintain a database of funding bodies from different specialisms which is updated on a regular basis. Information is disseminated to our Faculty by email circulars or in the staff bulletin, and email alerts can be set up.

Who can help?

The university's external projects team not only helps to find potential sources of money, they also offer help and advice to support the bid-writing process. As an expert in your own field of work you will understand the context of the bid, but writing bids is a skill in its own right and training or help from experienced writers who understand how each submission is put together should be welcomed in your early days.

Most organisations have someone responsible for human resources (HR), and every project needs people to make them happen. The HR department can give guidance and support on policies and procedures appropriate to employing staff in your organisation. As you prepare your bid you will need to consider:

- the nature of the contracts of employment of project staff
- legal considerations relating to their employment
- the associated job descriptions, person specifications and salary scales.

Make sure, too, that they give permission for their names or information to be included in your bid documentation.

If your bid is successful you will want to start work on the project as quickly as possible, and if these HR issues have already been thought about and any problems solved, they are less likely to hold you up now. If you need to recruit new people to the team,

Case study A (continued)

Once the contract had been agreed in principle, the project leader and I met the contractors to agree the package they required from the three proposed funding strategies of our bid. I was warned prior to the meeting that the negotiations would be lively and challenging, and that it was important to make a full note of the interim decisions as items were agreed. This proved to be true and showed how important it was to be well prepared, and to understand the need to agree a price at which the budget covered all the dimensions of the work satisfactorily.

they will often have to work a notice period once appointed, unless they are to be seconded from another department or organisation. Project work by its very definition is a fixed-term activity, and it can often be a difficult decision to move from a permanent contract elsewhere into short-term contract work. They will want to know that the project has been well thought through, how long their contract will be, how long the project will last, what is the likelihood of continuing in your employment when the project and funding ceases, and the details of their terms and conditions (for example, their rights to study leave and protected time for development).

Involve your organisation's finance department at an early stage of the bid preparation. Look at Chapter 5 to see the multitude of issues to consider when drawing up the budget. Final negotiations will take place once the contract has been agreed in principle, but before then you need to be realistic about what you can achieve for the costings you specify, and about how much 'give and take' there can be between yourselves and the commissioning body.

What do you bid for?

Do you jump in and look for big contracts, or do you start small? Within a university, staff often bid for contracts as part of their role in research, enterprise or teaching. It is important that you do not overstretch yourself so that you can continue to fulfil all of your commitments. However, if a large contract is announced about which you are enthusiastic and that you have the skills and knowledge to undertake, then it is worth putting a proposal together, either alone or with a consortium of staff.

By being selective about which sources of funding to go for when entering the 'competition', and perhaps by starting with small-scale projects, you can learn from your own experience and build up a new set of skills, while at the same time bringing new money into your organisation.

Research ethics considerations

Consider applying for research ethics approval once you have drawn up the project protocol and before funding is in place. Some funding bodies ask for ethical approval before they will consider a bid or release funding, and it is important to get the timing right of your submission to a research ethics committee (see page 39). Within our Faculty we have a director responsible for research and enterprise. All projects must be approved by the director prior to submission to an external research ethics committee or funding body.

Writing the bid

Work with others in your team to compile the bid. Pay particular attention to the nature of your role in the bid and any sections you are responsible for writing, but ensure these fit within the context of the whole document. We have found the following tips useful:

- Use an appropriate style of writing. Don't use jargon unless it is unavoidable; instead, use language that is clear, simple and to the point. If you have received a detailed tender document from the funding body/commissioner, consider adopting their style and approach.
- Do not waffle. Try to keep sentences to no more than twenty words, and make each sentence specific and succinct.
- Show your enthusiasm for the goals and content of the bid. Demonstrate your (or your team's) thorough knowledge and expertise in the funding area by addressing the bid requirements in a targeted way. Your experience and expertise in the bid areas must be highlighted with flair and innovation (if that style is appropriate to the nature of the proposal or funding body). We have achieved this through the information we have provided, and also by having appropriate 'expert' collaborators included in the bid.

We have attended workshops on writing for publication and workshops to share good practice in bidding for funds. Workshops and training sessions such as these are advertised at universities and teaching hospitals, or are offered by private-sector organisations or training bodies. The workshop at which we shared good practice was particularly valuable. Not only did we learn from colleagues' and others' experiences, we also shared our successful bidding documentation and tenders with each other. This helped us to highlight key success factors and illustrated the different approaches expected by particular funding bodies or commissioners. It was also a good opportunity to network and identify potential collaborators with similar interests and expertise for future bids.

Managing your time

If you are leading the construction of the proposal, managing your time effectively is vital if you are to produce a professional bid by the deadline. Make sure that all team members or contributors have time to review, revise, add comments, etc. Do not underestimate the time it takes to put together the bid documentation and send it in.

You should break down the bid preparation into specific tasks and set strict deadlines for completing each component. Ensure that these deadlines are realistic and that you communicate them to all the contributors. Allow time for contributors to read and review the documentation and any relevant background work that the funding bodies or you/your team have obtained. If possible, arrange a meeting of key team members at the start of the process, and then at appropriate stages before the proposal is finalised.

If meetings aren't feasible due to time or budgetary constraints, it might be possible to compile the bid by email, with the leader collating responses. If in doubt about any aspect of the bid documentation it's usually possible to send queries to the funding body or commissioner (the appropriate contact details are generally included in the initial documentation or invitation to tender). If you manage your time wisely, there should be no need to rush any aspect of completing the documentation unless there are unforeseen circumstances, such as sickness or a sudden crisis. If your instinct is that certain areas of the proposal look weak or insubstantial, take the time to reinforce those areas by the inclusion of research findings, key policies, statistics, etc.

Case study B describes a novice's perspective on compiling part of a tender submission. The importance of allowing sufficient time to write your part of a proposal is emphasised. You will see that, for those for whom bid writing is new, being honest both with yourself and others in the team about your capabilities, expertise and knowledge is key. If you are having difficulty with any part of the bidding process, seek training or guidance to give you the necessary knowledge or skills for making future bids or completing your current one if there is time. Could another member of the team take on this part of the task instead of you? If your uncertainty is due to inexperience within your organisation in a particular area or skill, do you know of an external collaborator you might involve, or could you bid with another organisation with the strengths you lack?

Case study B
(Sara Buckley)

The first time I was asked to contribute to writing a bid I felt flattered and excited to be included but unsure that I could fulfil the requirements placed upon me. Fortunately the project leader was experienced both in writing bids and in the subject area of the bid. My responsibility was to work up the project costings, prepare the necessary budget according to our organisational finance procedures, and obtain any necessary procedural statements from our organisation to include in the bid.

The bid documentation was quite complex and, in addition to the main content of the bid, it also required:

- detailed management arrangements for the project, including CVs and copies of qualifications and membership of professional bodies for each individual in the bidding team
- completion of several budget tables, including details of individual staff hours on the proposed project, invoice and finance details for our organisation, additional expenses and any discounts given for the volume of work undertaken annually
- measures taken to ensure excellent client care and how any conflicts that arose during the project would be managed
- details of procedures for dealing with complaints
- quality assurance details for our organisation.

As I was to project manage the proposed project if we were successful in our bid, it was my responsibility to provide this information and to follow the correct procedures to send off our submission. With clear leadership, I knew what my tasks were and, critically, that I could ask for help if I could not complete, or had difficulty with, any of these tasks. This was crucial, as time was short; and if I looked as if I would be unable to complete them it was important for the success of the bid that I asked for help in good time.

continued

Case study B (continued)

Information was difficult to find for some components of the bid. Though I was fortunate to work for a large organisation with access to personnel, finance and other support services, and with a website bearing details of policies and procedures, it was still difficult to find some specific information. The main problems were ensuring that the information I found was up to date, succinct and relevant. I had great help from colleagues who either had previous experience of bid-writing or could introduce me to those who had.

I passed the information to the project leader to disseminate amongst the team, so that any amendments to the proposal could be made in good time. I allowed time in my diary to thoroughly check the bid requirements against our submission to make sure that we had answered all the questions posed and provided all of the information requested. Time was again allocated in my diary for a final check of the submission (that we had enclosed the correct number of paper copies, etc.) and to ensure that we had completed all the requirements, before submitting our bid.

Then we just had to wait to hear if we had been shortlisted.

Tips for attending an interview

If your bid is successful and you are shortlisted, you may be asked to attend an interview before the final award decision is made. Allow sufficient time to prepare for the interview, and take care in choosing the presenting team. The funding body should outline what you can expect in the interview: the length of time of the interview, details of any presentation you may be expected to give (the availability of audiovisual equipment, etc.). If you need more details, contact them to obtain this information.

A copy of the presentation may be required in advance, but even if this is the case, take an electronic back-up copy with you and print out good-quality paper copies to leave for the interview team. It may sound obvious, but also take with you the contact details of the person arranging the interview and a map of the general location of the venue you are attending. Then if you are delayed you can let them know in advance. On one occasion we were notified of a venue change on the morning of the presentation, and had an anxious thirty minutes trying to find the venue, get there on time, and notify another team member who was travelling separately. From this experience we would recommend taking the mobile phone numbers of any other presenters who are travelling separately from you. Ideally all of the presenting team should have sufficient knowledge of each others' contributions to be able to substitute for them if necessary.

Top interview tips for someone new to the bidding process are:

- Find out as much as you can about the interview panel. Find out how many people will be present. and who they are. Take the time to research their backgrounds so that you gain insights into both the types of question they may ask and the responses that may interest or enthuse them.
- Coordinate the presentation coherently so that there is a clear flow of information, and each presenter contributes to the overall delivery of the proposal.
- Take along any background material you feel may be relevant, and decide beforehand if you will leave this with the interview panel whilst they make their decision.
- Project confidence at the interview. If you are well prepared and have confidence in your bid, ensure that this is clearly demonstrated. Agree a system for answering questions; the leader can delegate questions to the team, and each member will have specific responsibility for questions about 'their' part of the project.
- Prepare well in advance, practise the delivery of your presentation, anticipate likely questions and plan model answers. If possible the presenting team could plan a mock presentation to run through the process and help build their confidence.
- Do not assume that all of the interview panel will have thoroughly read your proposal. Outline the key facets in your presentation and refer to relevant sections where appropriate when answering questions. Keep your answers focused and succinct, clear, and where possible free from abbreviations and jargon.

The final tip in the above list arose from an unsuccessful bid application we made. We wrote a good research proposal and were shortlisted to attend for interview. The presentation we delivered focused on key aspects of the bid, but did not go into detail about the proposed research methodology. We assumed the panel members would have thoroughly considered this part of our documentation when shortlisting us and preparing their questions for us. During the interview it became apparent that this was not the case, and there was some confusion as we kept clarifying our approach. Though the feedback we obtained after-

Case study A (continued)

We were invited to present our bid to the national committee of the commissioning body in London. Whilst I had given presentations at conferences to both large and small groups, this was the first time I had been challenged and questioned in great detail about how a project proposal could be fulfilled. As the project leader was experienced, I was able to act in a supporting role. Together with the proposed contracts manager, we gave a PowerPoint presentation. We explained how we would tackle the project in a structured manner. The project leader delivered the bulk of the presentation, while each team member present one PowerPoint slide to contribute to the overall delivery of the presentation.

When we entered the room I was surprised at the number of people on the interview panel; about fifteen altogether. We were given an hour to present our bid and to answer any questions that arose. Questions were asked both during and after the presentation, so it was important that we all had a good understanding of the project and our limitations. Our project leader fielded most of the questions.

The whole process was both exhausting and invigorating at the same time. The questions were searching, and it was necessary to think quickly in a stressful environment in order to give the client a clear indication of what we as a team could deliver. We wanted to show that our proposed product was the best solution for them. It was nerve wracking, and I remember coming out of the meeting unsure about whether we would be given the contract.

I have learnt from this experience that you must identify what you can and cannot do before attending the interview. Whilst it is important to maintain some flexibility in what you are willing to do, there is no point offering the earth if you know you will be unable to fulfil the contract. Each member of the presenting team needs to be familiar with the proposed project, and to work together in the interview situation. We needed to be well prepared as a presenting team, and confident that we would each answer in a similar way if asked.

wards did not highlight this aspect of our performance at the interview, our lack of clarity could only have been detrimental to our chances of success.

Celebrating success and coping with disappointment

Feedback should be obtained whether you are successful or not. This will help you to learn more about success factors and gain insights from your experience of bidding. Do not be put off if you are unsuccessful; the knowledge you gain along the way will invariably be useful, and the successes – when they do come – will make it all worthwhile. Use what you learn from your experiences to action plan for future bids.

Reference

1   Natarajan A. Research for beginners. *BMJCareers*. 2006; 1 July: gp9.

Chapter 9

Learning the lessons

Ruth Chambers

Inform your co-bidders or collaborators of the outcome of your bid as soon as possible, whether or not you have been successful – you don't want them to hear from someone else first. Debrief your team after the whole process is over, and learn what you could do better next time.

Some lessons you might draw on

Many of these 'lessons' have been described in earlier chapters of this book, but they bear repetition; and even those experienced at making bids or submitting tenders need to be reminded about most of these pointers.

- Draw on the expertise or help available from any expert resource relating to research and development, innovation or enterprise in your organisation.
- Be familiar with your organisation's current business plan or new drafts; this will underpin your pursuit of external consultancy and other work.
- Understand the varying amounts of overheads your organisation charges for different types of external work. Where these are not permitted by a funding body, e.g. by charitable organisations, then take hard decisions about tendering.
- Do not confront those in public-sector organisations with blanket overhead charges in your bid or tender. Itemise costings as distinct expenses, so they can see what they would be paying for.
- Be selective about which tenders or bids you go for. Invest your energy in bids where you have a good chance of succeeding.
- Try to involve other experts in your organisation or in collaborating organisations to pull together tenders; but when inviting others be specific about their role/experience and likely input; avoid general 'meetings' where individuals cannot prioritise their attendance and senior people may be absent.

- Only prepare and submit a bid or tender if you have time to do it justice.
- Relate your bid or tender to any underpinning NHS or social care national policies, to match what you perceive to be the sponsor's aims even if they are poorly expressed in the funding body's documentation.
- Set up an 'intelligence' network in your organisation so that you know of future tenders or awards before they are announced; get on the tendering list of local/national organisations.
- Speak to those inviting the tender as much as is relevant – don't guess what they want if it's not clear. Within the bounds of professional behaviour, use the opportunity to sell your ideas before submitting the tender, so the sponsor understands what you're contributing.
- When writing a tender or bid, try to get an electronic copy of the invitation (or procurement) document and insert answers/solutions for each component. That helps one submitted bid or tender to be compared with another; and your good value be demonstrated.
- Contextualise the bid or tender you are submitting. You need to know exactly what the sponsors want before submitting it (from market intelligence, previous contacts, internet, national policies, colleagues' experience).
- You need 'off-the-shelf' contracts that you can adapt when you are successful in relation to a particular bid.
- Coordinate the bidding activity in your organisation and be aware of what each other is doing and bidding for, so that you do not find out later that you are competing against a colleague.
- Acknowledge the effort and preliminary work that needs to be done before a successful bid can start.
- Look back and review any evaluations of you or your partners' previous work – their track record, quality, value for money – from the commissioners' perspectives. Then revise your next tender or bid to those organisations accordingly.

Communicating your research or project results widely

As soon as your project gets under way you should be considering what to do with the findings. The essential element in undertaking research or establishing a new initiative is letting others know about your findings – positive or negative. So you need to disseminate news about your methods and results in research papers or reports that are good enough to be published in internationally acclaimed peer-reviewed journals, or in the core publications of high-profile national organisations. Seminars, workshops and conference presentations are the way the academic community shares research findings, discusses results and challenges each others' work. Books and articles and teaching materials may develop research or evaluation findings further, setting the programme of work in context or applying it in creative ways.

If you are the team leader you will encourage your team members to learn these communication and dissemination skills, so that gradually they lead on the writing of the papers or reports or presenting the results in other ways, planning and delivering workshops and contributing to influential conferences.

Making the most of a poster display

Think of your work on a poster at a conference and see it as the opportunity for a two-way exchange of information between you and those looking at the poster. Target your audience so that the poster is written in the right language, with messages that are important to them and in a style they expect. Remain focused so that the key messages are clear and not lost in a lot of unnecessary text.

Make the findings or recommendations clear, using simple graphs that are easy to comprehend in a short time. Stand beside your poster at breaks in the conference, or put your contact details on the poster (mobile phone number/email address) so that you can meet up at the conference or communicate afterwards. If there is an opportunity to talk about your work for a few minutes while standing next to your poster, take it, even if it inconveniences you. Leave handouts containing your contact details in plastic pockets attached to the poster (not on the floor where they can get kicked about or where people cannot be bothered to bend down to pick one up). Take sufficient handouts with you – it might be difficult or expensive to photocopy more at the conference venue.

When you're back in your own organisation, display your poster on the wall of a corridor or meeting room to maximise the promotion of your work and achievements.

Addressing under-performance in your team

Under-performance can cover a range of issues, such as people's knowledge, skills, behaviour and attitudes. As a leader you should have created systems to diagnose, assess and support those for whom you are responsible, in your immediate team or beyond, who are under-performing. Under-performance is about achieving less than expected, or performing below required levels or explicit standards. Sometimes under-performance is defined in terms of consistently behaving in a way that generates risk.

Individuals who under-perform:

- may be generally passive
- may find challenge frightening and avoid it whenever possible
- may lack insight about their shortcomings
- may find feedback and criticism threatening
- may have low reserves of energy
- may have poor motivation
- may resent others' success
- may fail to realise their potential.

Sometimes the problem arises from a malfunctioning organisation, such as:

- poor management of quality processes
- inadequate infrastructure and insufficient resources to undertake tasks
- poor communication within the work setting
- an unhealthy culture within the organisation
- a culture of fear and lack of openness
- a lack of leadership, or inappropriate styles of management and organisational structure.

Whatever the cause, learn the lessons from any recent or current work you have been doing in which one or more of those working for you have under-performed; and set up a new approach to prevent under-performance, or at least to detect and then deal with it as early as possible.

How to make enemies without really trying

Here are some actions and circumstances you won't want to reproduce!

- Put in a bid, or publish research with your name as author, without including the names and contributions of others who have contributed vision, ideas and effort.
  So: be inclusive and remember to acknowledge everyone who has contributed.
- Plagiarise others' ideas or work without acknowledging the

source (obviously this is illegal and unprofessional, but in small amounts it is difficult to prove, while at the early stages of developing a project proposal or bid, the initial thinking is easily borrowed).

So: do not plagiarise, even in small degrees, unintentionally or otherwise.

- Attend a networking meeting or give a presentation without acknowledging others' contributions fully.

  So: remember those acknowledgements even when you're under time pressures or otherwise feeling stressed.

- Disagree in your assessment of various people's contributions and individuals' perspectives.

  So: get initial agreement or understanding of who will lead on what aspect.

- Insist, require or expect that, as the senior member of the team, your name will go first or nearly first in the order of authors' names in a conference abstract, published paper, research proposal or bid (especially when others dare not 'cross' you in case this has an impact on their future support or personal references).

  So: use national recommended best practice in deciding the order of authors' names.

- As leader of an organisation or a collaborative group, take all offers of help and input whilst putting together a research or project bid, but once funding is agreed shut out the collaborators and distribute funding and prestigious opportunities unfairly, or keep collaborators in the dark about development of the project – or even fail to notify collaborators about progress with the bid so that the first they hear about the success of the bid or other related achievements is via the media.

  So: be honest and straightforward with collaborators; make agreements about how the project will be actioned and funding shared at initial planning meeting; draw up official an memorandum.

- Engage in dubious and/or unethical practices when pursuing research or project protocol, so that you also tarnish other people's names and reputations.

  So: know what constitutes unethical practice and don't do it.

- Disparage other people connected with your project or research in a public forum, or in a supposedly private and confidential discussion from which someone might your remarks.

  So: be honest, fair and straightforward, respecting other contributors and your allies.

- Make it clear what 'Chatham House Rules' means, but do not trust such an agreement to be upheld if you do make defamatory comments.

  So: don't make such comments!

- Disparage senior or influential people, or cast doubt upon their commitment, expertise or reliability, whether or not you know them; either because you have any substantial information or you are merely voicing your frustration at their possession of power or influence or casting doubt about their commitment, expertise or reliability.

  So: watch what you say or imply; give credit and praise where it is due; make factual and objective remarks rather than give subjective opinions.

- Undertake or plan to carry out 'research' without applying for or obtaining research ethics or research governance approval; and wrongly term your work a 'survey' or 'audit'. Reputable journals will refuse to publish a report of the work.

  So: know the regulations about research ethics and research governance and adhere to them.

- Ignore best practice in equality and diversity, thus perhaps discriminating against people in relation to their gender, age, discipline, disability, ethnicity, etc., whether knowingly or unknowingly. Witnesses who do nothing (and feel guilty about not tackling or confronting you), and sufferers (who seemingly ignore or tolerate your behaviour), will dislike you, feel angry or victimised, and criticise you. They may make a formal complaint about your discriminatory behaviour.

  So: adhere to best practice in equality and diversity, and adopt practical measures to demonstrate thoughtfulness to others promotion of equal opportunities.

- Promise to complete an activity as part of the bid or project and then neglect or ignore it, especially if it is a critical component and you do not flag up your omission, or worse, you pretend to be doing something when you aren't.

  So: go on a time-management course, or, better still, put what you learn or already know about good time management into practice.

- Drive others (e.g., your research team) too hard against unrealistic deadlines or towards unachievable goals, and then blame them (perhaps publicly) for not meeting those deadlines or goals – especially when the lack of time and resources is obvious, there is an excess of competing priorities or a lack of skills and training.

So: be realistic when planning the proposal and subsequent work programme from start to finish, and allow for unpredictable events.

- Lie, cheat, have tantrums or generally misbehave.
  So: give yourself a makeover.
- Put someone's name on a bid, a report or a paper, or nominate them as a referee, without asking them first.
  So: remember your manners.
- As part of a commissioning body considering tenders, leak the details of a particular tender – resources, costs, capacity – to a competitor, so that the competitor could take advantage of that information when putting future competitive bids.
  So: take your responsibility for confidentiality seriously.
- Abuse your position as a peer reviewer, perhaps stealing the ideas from a paper or grant application which you are reviewing for your own ends, meanwhile criticising the paper or grant application so that it is turned down or returned for amendments.
  So: be objective; be aware if there may be a conflict of interest, and step down from being a peer reviewer in that instance.

Chapter 10

And finally: how to make sure that your proposal is rejected

Elizabeth Boath

Now that you have read through the previous nine chapters and realised what a tremendous amount of work is involved in conceiving, then preparing and submitting a bid or proposal, let alone doing the work if you are successful, you might want to make sure that you are not awarded the funding. Here's how.

You're only as good as your proposal, so there is nothing as effective as a poorly written, ill-conceived proposal to convince reviewers that the methodology is unsound and that you have little grasp of the literature or major issues in the field and so will be completely incompetent at carrying out the proposed work. Then you will not have all the work to do that comes with a successful bid.

Instructions

First (and the most essential step), put any instructions about the bidding process straight in the bin. Do not under any circumstances be tempted to read them. If you do succumb to reading them, then be sure to:

- ignore the word count requirement (they'll never check) and make your submission of epic proportions
- ignore the questions that the sponsors want answered and turn them into those that you want to answer instead
- ensure that your proposal arrives late, well past the closing date; if it's good enough they're bound to wait for it. They should realise that someone as busy and highly sought after as you is worth waiting for.
- Put the wrong address on, or address your submission to the wrong person (and don't forget to mis-spell their name and get their gender wrong) to test their systems.

Layout

- Handwritten proposals are great (it adds a personal touch as well as being impossible to read).
- Submit on loose-leaf paper and include more than the requested number of pages.
- Cross out words and leave gaps in the text.
- Make sure that there is no structure to your proposal.
- Forget about getting everyone to sign the bid. So long as your signature is on it, what more can they want or expect?

Abstract

This is the summary or framework for your proposed work. Reviewers will read this first, and may make an instant decision based on it. So, to ensure rejection:

- Don't leave it until last to write it. Instead, write it straight away and off the top of your head; it's your project after all.
- Make sure that you do not include the planned work/research question, the rationale for the work, the hypothesis, or the methodology to be used (e.g., the design, the procedures, the participants and any instruments).
- Do go into irrelevant detail.

Title

- Make it vague, cute, long-drawn-out, ambiguous and uninformative.
- Include meaningless phrases such as 'An investigation of…'.
- Don't worry about including independent and dependent variables.
- Include as many multi-syllabic words as possible to impress the panel.

References

- If it says five references maximum (they really mean 10), the more the better.
- Don't cite seminal papers and do cite irrelevant or trivial references instead. They should be familiar with the seminal papers anyway if they know their stuff.
- Rely on secondary sources.
- Don't check that references are complete and correct. That

should keep them on their toes.

- Don't be consistent about the reference style; a mixture of Vancouver, Harvard and your own made-up styles will suffice. Alternatively, copy the example of this chapter and give no references whatsoever; then they will know the content of your bid is all your own original work.

Language

Make sure you use:

- jargon and colloquialisms
- trendy words and 'in' phrases
- abbreviations and acronyms (without explaining them in full; it will seem impressive that you use these terms as part of your everyday language)
- spelling errors, typos and grammatical errors
- alternative spellings from other countries, which give you a worldly air
- language that does not reflect that of the sponsors, so you are not writing for your 'audience', in case it looks as if you were toadying to them.

Background/ introduction

Do not under any circumstances:

- cite previous, recent, ongoing or unpublished work in the field, as this may suggest to sponsors that you know a lot about what you are proposing
- waste time keeping up with recent developments
- critically evaluate cited papers
- provide a context to frame the proposed work
- accurately present theoretical and empirical contributions by other researchers.
- stay focused on the planned work
- develop a persuasive and coherent argument for the planned work.

Methods

The key thing about the methodology section is that it should provide detailed plans of what you propose to do. So, to make sure that your proposal is rejected:

- make the description of your methods vague and provide very

little information on what you plan to do.
- do not state whether you will take a qualitative or quantitative approach, or a combination of both; let the panel work that out for themselves.
- do not describe measurement tools or the reasons for your choice. There's no need to provide evidence of their reliability and validity either.
- do not include details about the participants, e.g. their age, gender, ethnicity, etc., or of how you will access them and what sampling procedure you will use. That will leave your options open once you get going on the project, at which point you can judge what level of bias you can get away with.
- do not provide justification of your choice of method over and above other methods; if the funding body has the right expertise to judge your bid, they should be able to compare your chosen methodology with other possibilities.

Participants

Do not:

- specify exactly who the subjects will be
- state the inclusion or exclusion criteria
- demonstrate that you have access to the participants and that they are likely to support the proposed work; you wouldn't be proposing to recruit the subjects if you didn't think there was a good chance of them cooperating, would you?
- mention that patients or potential participants have been involved in designing the proposal; after all, their lay opinions might be considered inferior to those of real professionals
- divulge much about the subjects you propose to recruit; if the funding agency has no knowledge of, or interest in, your participants, they won't pinch your subjects for similar work of their own.

Results

Obviously you do not have any results at this stage, so make some up. However, you need to have some idea about what kind of data you will be collecting, and what statistical procedures will be used in order to answer your research question or test your hypothesis. Sounds difficult? It's not. Just make that lot up too! It's easy. You read about research fraud all the time; the trick is not to get found out.

Discussion

It is important to convince the panel of the potential impact of your proposed research or project. You need to communicate a sense of enthusiasm and confidence without exaggerating the merits of your proposal. So don't bother to mention the potential limitations and weaknesses of the proposed work; they will never guess. By the time they find out, the funding will have been agreed and transferred and it will be too late for them to do anything about it. Your lack of progress then may be justified by time and financial constraints as well as by the early developmental stage of your research area.

Evaluation

- Do not mention how you will evaluate whether (or not, in this case!) your project has successfully achieved its objectives. Most people don't bother with evaluation, so why should you?
- Don't worry about the sustainability of the project. When the funding ends, so does your interest in it – unless you really have proved something important that more sponsors clamour to fund. Well, you can dream!

Project team

Think of all the reasons why you, your team and your organisation are uniquely placed to carry out the proposed work (expertise in relation to the topic, previous work in the field, close relationships with proposed participants, geographic location, etc.), but do not mention them. Simple as that. Other essential routes to failure include:

- Do not bother to get the right team on board. They will only get pregnant or become sick anyway and go off on leave.
- Do not bother to introduce them with formalities such as name, title, qualifications or experience. You don't need them when you're all equal.
- Do not clarify how each person contributes to the overall proposal. You might change your mind when you see what your staff are capable of, and designations could be restrictive.
- Do not bother forming a steering group (made up of experts, members of key organisations, etc.). That way you can save time by omitting the descriptions of members' roles, duration, etc.,

and save costs because there's no need to pay for those 'fat cat' lunches and boozy sessions.

Time line

There is nothing like showing a nice graphic to break up the tedium of your bid. Having not worked out exactly what you plan do, with whom you plan to do it, or when, drawing up a timeline or Gannt chart for the proposed work will be a simple piece of imagination; so:

*   do not state how long the proposed work will take
*   do make your graphic as complicated as you can
*   bamboozle the panel with your 'science'.

Resources, equipment and consumables

*   Make your budget as unrealistic as you can. Stick a finger in the air, or just think of a number between 1 and 10 and multiply it by £10,000 – or an even larger amount. That will probably be more accurate than slaving over a calculator to predict and gauge exact costs.
*   Your budget must not add up, let alone balance. The funding body's finance department will help out there.
*   Recruit lots of personnel, the more the merrier (don't forget to forget National Insurance and inflationary and incremental increases in salary).
*   Consultants can be very expensive and very unnecessary, so add them in. They will make your employing organisation see your own in-house staff as cheap in comparison when you make future bids.
*   Even if you are proposing quantitative work, add in unnecessary items such as a tape recorder, video, TV, etc. (for in-house office entertainment, of course, unless you've got them already; in which case, you can always take them home).
*   Successful bids are a good opportunity to get some new laptops, PCs, printers, desks, chairs, lamps and other office equipment, so the sky's the limit.
*   Even if you will get things for free, e.g. room space, cost them in.
*   Don't mention matched funding from other partner organisations; that way you end up with a nice little hidden surplus.
*   Add in the cost of tea and biscuits (chocolate ones essential) for

everyone, especially if your employing organisation normally expects you to buy such things yourself.
- When you're successful, ask for all the funding up front and not in phases (then you can spend it before the weaknesses in your bid are exposed).
- Whatever you do, do not pass your draft bid to your finance department for review. They might spot your 'deliberate' mistakes and not realise they are intentional.

Appendices

- This is an excellent opportunity to add lots of irrelevant pieces of paper, e.g. newsletters, presentations, handouts, etc. A nice bulky submission will impress the judges, who rarely read submissions all the way through anyway.
- Use generic letters of support; these will save you bothering your referees each time you bid.
- Include copies of every questionnaire or tool you might use, so they have them all to hand.

Ignore this at your peril!

Following the above advice will be a fantastic way of using up lots of time, so you'll never be bored. Then again, you'll never get any funding either. Failing to follow her own top tips has resulted in the author of this chapter obtaining more than £100,000 worth of funding in the last six months. So now she'd better go and do some real work!

Index